The Rosen Method of Movement

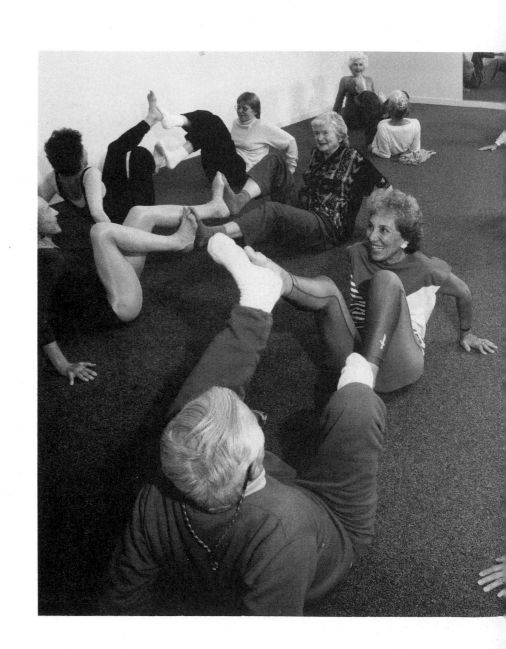

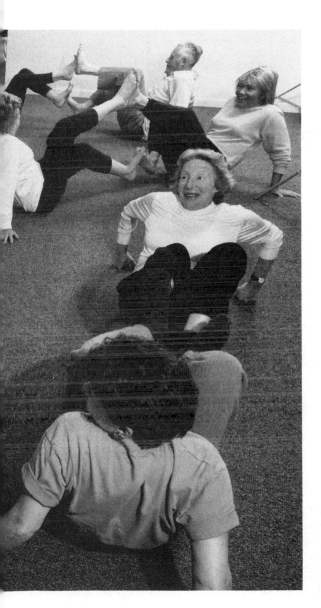

The Rosen Method of Movement

Marion Rosen & Sue Brenner

Illustrated by Jane Strong
Photographs by Paul Johnson

North Atlantic Books
Berkeley, California

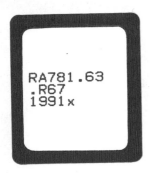
The Rosen Method of Movement

Published by
North Atlantic Books
2800 Woolsey Street
Berkeley, California 94705

Cover photo and book design by Paula Morrison

Printed in the United States of America

The Rosen Method of Movement is sponsored by the Society for the Study of Native Arts and Sciences, a nonprofit educational corporation whose goals are to develop an educational and crosscultural perspective linking various scientific, social, and artistic fields; to nurture a holistic view of arts, sciences, humanities, and healing; and to publish and distribute literature on the relationship of mind, body, and nature.

Library of Congress Cataloging-in-Publication Data

Brenner, Sue, 1950-
    The Rosen method of movement / by Sue Brenner and Marion Rosen.
      p.   cm.
    ISBN 1-55643-117-1 (pbk.) : $12.95
    1. Stretching exercises. 2. Breathing exercises. 3. Mind and Body.
  I. Rosen, Marion, 1914- . II. Title.
  RA781.63.B74 1991
  613.7--dc20
                                         91-35742
                                          CIP

Acknowledgments

Thanks to Marion's dancing ladies for their thirty years of dedication and inspiration, all the Rosen Method of Movement teachers for their ideas and support, Irene Meyers for helping to get the book started, Murray Brenner for babysitting the kids, Rusty Miller for his patience and computer knowledge, and Lindy Hough for her excellent editing.

Disclaimer

The reader must carefully apply the exercises and their underlying principles to his or her personal condition, using caution and common sense.

The book is designed to provide enough information to enable the reader to learn and do Rosen Movement safely.

This book is sold with the understanding that the publisher and authors are not engaged in rendering medical or other professional health services via the book and its contents. The purpose of this book is to educate and encourage the reader toward self-education. A health professional should be consulted for questions or problems. The authors and publisher have no liability or responsibility to any person or entity with respect to any loss, damage, or injury caused or alleged to be caused directly or indirectly by the information contained in this book.

No portion of this book may be reprinted without permission of the authors.

Preface

Students come to the class having heard of it by word of mouth. They have heard that Rosen Work is not just exercise; it is something that 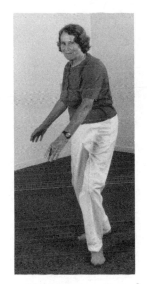 will make them feel different afterwards. They also see how their friends have changed. Students have the awareness that they can do something with the movement. The student begins to feel something internally. This is the difference between a work in and a work out. Timing that allows you to become aware of the impact of movement on the inside of the body is very different from mindless performed movement.

Our goal is to make people feel happy and motivated to dance rather than drag themselves around. We would like them to feel physically well when their bodies move, and emotionally cheerful. When people leave the class, they skip and dance, talking to each other. They laugh as they leave. They can often be heard saying, "I feel so good now!" and that is the result we like to have happen when people come to our class. One of the participants has said, "I enjoy your exercises because there is a physiological change in me when I do them," and this is true too. So we want people to be happy and feel good, and this is built on a very deep knowledge of anatomy and how people can move. We train people to know how to bring about this kind of freedom through movement.

Marion Rosen
Sue Brenner

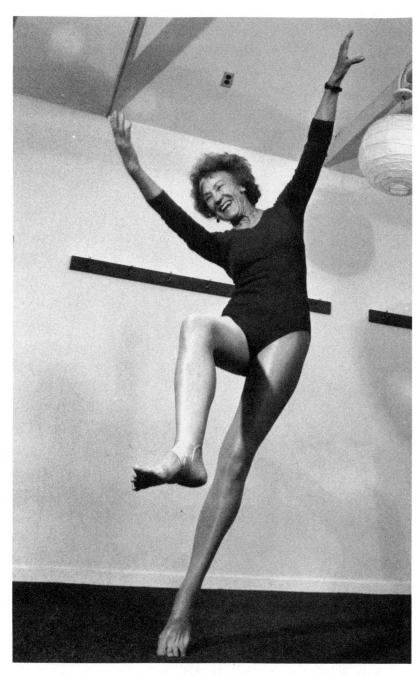

Joyful dancing at seventy-three years old.

Contents

CONTENTS

CONTENTS

Marion Rosen

Marion Rosen is a physical therapist born in Germany in 1914. While awaiting a visa to the U.S. in Sweden, she spent many hours observing dance classes. When she arrived in the United States a year and a half later, she realized she had learned from watching dance how a body moves: what a normal, full movement looked like as opposed to inhibited movement. Uninhibited movement looked wonderful, and it was something she loved to watch.

She had taken movement classes from the time she was seven from a local dance teacher. These classes were the highlight of Marion Rosen's week. "It was the most wonderful thing to go to her class because the teacher started out slowly, and there was always good music. She had a pianist to accompany us who would follow our movement while we danced. It was a totally satisfying experience, not only for us as children, but really for everybody who came there."

At school, however, she experienced very harsh movement and exercises, and she attended a class she hated that involved holding certain positions. She also noticed that no change occurred in the students afterwards. It was then she realized there was a real difference in the way movement is used, and what did and did not work.

Between 1936 and 1938 Rosen studied with Lucy Heyer, a pupil of Else Gindler, grandmother of today's breathing and relaxation techniques. Heyer's work was influenced by Mary Wigman in dance; Medau, the originator of a movement school using medicine balls; and Rudolf Laban, father of Laban Notation. She was a student of Jung and treated patients in breath, movement, and massage. Her husband, Dr. Gustav Heyer, treated the same patients with Jungian analysis. Heyer's classes loosened up patients to make their emotions more accessible to them.

Thus the pre-war German psychiatric circles influences on Rosen stressed the integration of physiologic and psychological analysis, as well as movement and breath work.

In 1938, while her brother was interning in psychiatry at the Tavstock Clinic in England, Rosen treated psychiatric patients with breath, massage, and bodywork. The results were excellent and many patients lost their symptoms.

After taking formal training in physical therapy in Sweden in the 1940's, Rosen repeated her training at the Mayo Clinic in the United States. She moved to Oakland, California and began a private practice. A friend asked her how to *prevent* aches and pains so that she could avoid having physical therapy treatments. This question inspired Rosen to begin teaching movement classes in 1956. She thought about all the exercises she had given private patients because they got stiff, because they had pain, because they couldn't move, and then organized a class around these same exercises as prevention against inability to move. It was "physical therapy in reverse."

When Marion Rosen began classes on her own, she gave her students time to breathe with the movements. She included not only simple movements, but also a combination of movements. She encouraged her physical therapy patients to attend the exercise classes as a way to avoid reinjury and to stay limber. Recognizing that music and rhythm were essential adjuncts to movement and that music could actually *make* people move, she set the exercise sequences to music. She came to understand through her classes that rhythm as well as moving in time with the music can be rehabilitating. She noticed that the bodies of her students stayed young, and that as they aged they could continue to perform the movements as easily, even better, than they did 33 years ago. Some of her students are between 70 and 83. They exercise only 45 minutes, once per week, and do not exercise otherwise, but they lead very active lives.

Chapter 1

Background Theory
of Rosen Work: Movement
and Bodywork

The Rosen Work concentrates on a process of relaxation whereby people allow themselves to release held muscles in their bodies. Relaxation is used as a gateway to awareness.

When we are not relaxed, we tighten certain areas of the body. Holding is contraction of a muscle, a muscle that works and has forgotten not to work. When a muscle is working, it shortens; when it is not working, it lengthens, i.e., it relaxes. A much different condition exists in a body when a muscle is contracted than when it is relaxed. Visualize what would happen to the body if all your muscles contracted simultaneously. Visualize all the muscles that go from top to bottom. If all these muscles were to contract, your body would shrink! You would be smaller. If the muscles around you from side to side were to contract, you would be narrower.

By releasing the muscle, you create more space. The space you create for yourself is the space you should be able to allow yourself to function in. The basic idea about health, in fact, is that you allow yourself the space you require to function in, no more and no less. When the space you work in is the space you are supposed to have, your organs can function the way they were meant to. However, people narrow their physical, emotional and mental range. Your diaphragm, for example, can swing the way a diaphragm was built to swing. When you allow the diaphragm to extend as far as it needs to go, then it opens your breathing space and supplies sufficient oxygen for the body's needs.

Breathing has a tremendous influence on the workings of the heart. The function of the heart is to distribute oxygen in the body. If very little oxygen is supplied with every breath, the heart must work faster and harder to supply oxygen to other parts of the body. The more oxygen per breath, the easier it is for the heart to operate. As the diaphragm swings up and down, the entire interior of the trunk, all of the body's organs, are continuously massaged and worked by the movement of the diaphragm. This steady movement is necessary for the body to function with ease.

Many people come for Rosen work—both movement and bodywork—because of a physical complaint or ailment. When a teacher and practitioner begins to work with a person, the teacher and practitioner can recognize areas where the student and client does not allow the breath to come in. Most students and clients will be satisfied when the pain goes away. For many people this is the end product. But some people want to go further to learn how to keep from having pain. This is where our work can make a difference.

Habit Patterns

As we grow from infancy to adulthood, we bring with us ways of functioning influenced by our life experiences. We call these habit patterns. Our lived experiences and our emotional responses to these experiences lead us into physical habit patterns that actually become *holding* patterns. These forms of habitual holding are what we work with in the Rosen Method.

Most of the work addresses reactions to experiences that could *not* be handled at the time they occurred and so were suppressed. Both the physical and the emotional state that existed at the time the experience was repressed are still there, but unavailable to the person who holds them. We store all our experiences and our reactions in our bodies. Inside our physical bodies are our mother's admonitions. "Pull yourself together! Don't make a fuss about it!" or "Don't yell! Be quiet! Shut up!" We may often have an impulse to shout but will inhibit the impulse because we've been told it is unacceptable behavior. We do not realize we have inhibited the healthy impulse however, and so when we get angry we feel anger build, and tighten those muscles that inhibit our yelling. This inhibiting response is based on tensing muscles, and becomes a habit pattern we engage in so repeatedly that it becomes automatic. Thus whenever something happens to trigger our anger, we immediately respond by inhibition through muscle contraction. While the reason for the habit pattern's formation has been long forgotten, it is still carried in the subconscious. We are not consciously aware that we behave the way we do because something specific happened to cause this kind of behavior. We simply take it at face value that this is who we are and how we function.

Habit patterns are also developed in response to trauma, manifesting in a survival syndrome. At some time or other each of us has had to pull ourselves together, to be brave; we may have been scared to death or may have had to be silent to survive danger.

People frequently confronted by survival situations manifest in their bodies the difficulties they have lived through in their lives. The goal of the Rosen work—movement and bodywork—is to help them determine what their lives would have been like if survival were not at stake. In the bodywork talking to clients is very important, as is working with the hands. In some instances the experiences that triggered the survival response surface in response to touch. Pain, sadness, loneliness, anger— all kinds of emotions may be released in response to contact with the worker's hands. Rather than get stuck in those feelings, the practitioner must make the client aware that these feelings are what were felt at the time the experience occurred. This is where the voice comes in. The purpose of talking in Rosen bodywork is to communicate what the practitioner perceives is occurring and relate it to the client.

As the client discovers what is real at that particular moment, she/he may realize that hiding may be inappropriate now. By letting more be revealed, the person may change the way he or she meets the world. We support each client's experience of meeting the world in a different way. By becoming aware, the individual can consider what other choices he or she may have. Perhaps the greatest benefit of the Rosen work—be it movement or bodywork—is its ability to bring people to the point of choosing different ways of expressing themselves—different ways of looking, of moving, of interacting.

This is the essence of the work. The movement teacher's exercises and the bodyworker's hands help a client release holdings, and bring the body into a way of being that permits expansion and mobility. The student is guided into finding out who he or she really is, what his or her potential is, and with that knowledge comes self-acceptance.

Relationship between Movement and Bodywork

Movement opens people up and facilitates the bodywork. If we relax when we move, we do not exert effort. Every movement comes from our center, our core. This way the whole body is involved with every movement. Sometimes in movement class emotions come up, yet we do not speak directly to them. People take the openness from bodywork or movement into their lives and carry it into the world. The openness from the exercise classes supports the bodywork. We use the freedom of our bodies, when we reach for dishes or sweep the floor, to make everyday life a dance. When we put our clothes on, we should

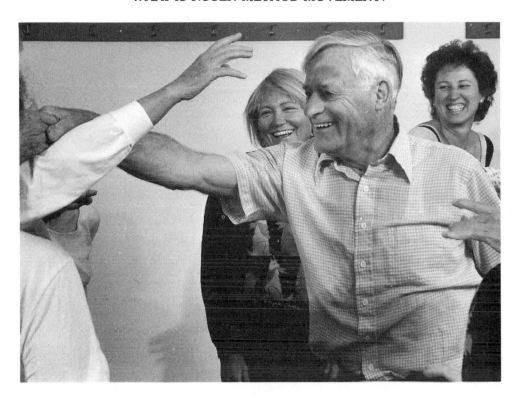

not use them as a shell, but instead let them reflect our openness. We teach physical awareness which reshapes the body through movement. The breath is a monitor both in movement and bodywork. When it is free, we know the participant can be fully present.

What is the Rosen Method of Movement?

In Rosen movement, healing manifests itself as a reclaiming of movements. The body begins to move again as a whole with the freedom of early childhood. Places long held frozen and unconscious are released. These stuck places are experienced as moving merely because they are no longer held.

For any of this to occur, the teacher must be moving with aliveness, an "inner wiggle." She or he must be an explorer, communicating

5

curiosity and joy in the student's new discoveries. To do this, the teacher must be alert to observing and affirming subtle differences and seeing the progress of the student toward fuller functioning.

The work is also based on the knowledge of the function of all joints. We work towards the student obtaining a full range of motion in every joint. The task in every class is to move every joint of the body by loosening the muscles around the joints. The tools are good music, simple movements and clear instructions. The movements include swings, stretches, bounces and twists.

The vital core and spirit of the Rosen Work is breath. The warm-up section of the class not only loosens the muscles and increases the range of motion, but also releases the diaphragm and increases the space in the chest for breath. The movements of the teacher and of the class ideally follow the expanding breath as it moves through the body. While following the breath, the body anticipates the next movement. The end of a class is marked by a joyful celebration of being together as whole individuals, which gives the class its very special energy.

Rosen Movement Objectives

* To move the joints systematically during each session so that fuller range of motion is potentiated. This joint lubricating is a prelude to any locomotion.

* To expand the chest and rib cage so that more breath can be taken in and the diaphragm freed.

* To lengthen muscles so that holding patterns can change and more room can be created for breathing fully.

* To focus on relaxation rather than moving with unnecessary effort, modifying habitual states of contraction.

* To reshape the body without hurting it

- To prepare the body for more strenuous activity.

- To re-educate participants on How to move without effort.

- To use movement to reach frozen, stiff or blocked places.

- To increase awareness of the interconnection of areas of the body.

- To facilitate moving with joy and ease in new ways.

- To use repetition and simplicity in movement for accessibility and fun.

- To build complex sequences upon simpler ones.

- To pause during a class in order to let participants notice breath and feeling.

- To teach letting go—not holding back or being careful—using the body in a freer, less inhibited way.

- To increase a sense of balance and rhythm.

- To provide an amount of exercise adequate to maintain function and mobility even in older age.

- To serve as a preventative health tool.

- To teach students that tightness does not define them; that they have choices about how their body moves and feels.

Basic Theory

Rosen Movement is a system of range of motion and stretching exercises. These are designed to lubricate the joints, expand the chest, and loosen the diaphragm.

To encourage all class participants' interest in the movements Marion Rosen introduced the same movements but with variations and varied the sequence of her instructions. She understood that for people teaching the kind of motions she was using required knowledge of how the body works and what it can do when it is normal. Then it is possible to apply movements to rehabilitate areas of the body that are not moving.

Rosen Movement has two major themes: structure and movement. Structural positions are the norm for how the body should work. There are also positions from which the body does not work. Rosen Movement addresses its exercises to the structural positions. Exercises are done to promote movement of the joints in the full range position.

Muscles are the agents that move the joint, where the bones approximate each other. The exercises are designed to work the muscles: the joint is being worked by the muscle; the bones are being moved around the joints. We work to have the muscles in the best condition by *teaching them to release and contract.* Because so much of the time we contract our muscles, automatically and unconsciously, a good deal of Rosen Movement involves relaxation exercises. At the moment we release we can also contract. *To get full use of an exercise we have to relax first, and then contract.* If the body is being taught that, then it will go on doing that. With this as its guiding principle, Rosen Movement uses a great deal of swinging and stretching, moving the joints easily and improving body function. When the body is functioning, various movements are combined into more complex movements. The exercise routine starts with the very simplest movements—the arm up and down; forward and backwards, and continues with combinations of simple movements. When students become comfortable with these movements, they proceed at a faster pace with more complicated movements. The tempo of the exercises is slow at the beginning, but speeds up as the routine proceeds.

One of the major components of Rosen Meovement is its emphasis on awareness of simple to complex, slow to fast. There is always a constant flow of movement, not dwelling on any one movement for too long, so that *movements are done only so long as they are pleasurable.*

The joy that goes into the movement is what is important, not working the body to boredom or to exasperation.

We also consider the interaction between the class and teacher an integral part of the work. "I don't shut people up when they talk—unless it's too loud and I can't hear myself anymore," Rosen has said. Often classes are marked by laughter, which we consider a confirmation that the class "really starts to let go."

Music has always been a significant feature of the class. Especially important is the choice of music to play. Many types of music are used depending on the teacher's personal taste. Suggestions are given in the back of this book. We use both records and tapes depending on the equipment available. Tapes are smaller, and more portable to travel with. Different rhythms enhance the same simple movements, and give a totally different way of moving. A quality that stimulates the student's wish to move is the overriding factor in selecting music for the exercises. Music must support the movement. Thus, it is important to plan what music will be played about a half-hour before the class commences. It always has to be some music *we enjoy*.

Another feature of Rosen Movement is its emphasis on attention to people as they move. "It is very important that people know they are being watched during class," suggests Marion. Rather than criticize people if they are doing the movement incorrectly we stand in front of the students as they do the movement so they can follow what we are doing more closely. We praise students when they perform a movement correctly.

Pausing for breath is another significant feature of the Rosen class. When people move too fast from one movement to another, they hold their breath. We pause to change the music or rest between exercises to wait for the agitation to die down before starting again. We also plan a movement for the very end of the class that is more like a dance than an exercise, so that students can fully enjoy their looseness, move freely and use the space with their whole body.

The floor exercises primarily involve the *spine.* The spine requires a range of motion as much as other joints do, even if the movements are very small. Together the smaller movements comprise bigger movements. When the spine moves in all the directions it can move, the body has achieved what Marion Rosen calls *"joint function."*

Every Rosen Movement Class Includes:

Joint lubrication
Chest and rib expansion
Releasing the Diaphragm
Muscle lengthening
Relaxation
Reshaping the body
Preparation of the body for more strenuous movement

Joint Lubrication

When we do not move the joints once a day, the synovial fluid that greases joints diminishes and fails to lubricate the joints adequately. Sometimes when we are not moving, in order *not* to move we have to hold somewhere. The holding around the joint becomes unconscious, preventing the joint from being moved. After the joint has been inactive for a while, it becomes exceedingly difficult to move it again. This can be quite a painful process—particularly if it has progressed over a long time. Therefore, it is crucial to prevent a joint from becoming dry. Movement stimulates the production of synovial fluid in the joints. When students say their joints are cracking, that is a sign that a static area is beginning to loosen up.

In every class we include full range of motion for the major joints by performing: abduction (moving a limb away from the body); adduction (moving a limb towards the body); inward and outward rotation; flexion and extension. The result is that people experience all of the body's possibilities.

Every joint needs space. There must be space between the bones for the joint to move. If the muscles around the joint are tense, the space becomes smaller. The bones may rub together instead of clearing each other but when we relax the muscles around the joints or stretch them, space is recreated. Synovial fluid is again produced, and the joint can work in a healthy, non-painful way.

Chest and Rib Expansion

It is very important to give the chest the expansion it needs, and to give the diaphragm the possibility of swinging. The breath comes and goes if you don't hold it back. The exercises provide as much space as people need. Stretching affords the whole body more space. Shoulder movements and stretches are done at the beginning of class to allow for chest and rib expansion. Any movement that is done using the shoulder is itself a chest movement and also a movement that opens space for the diaphragm. People with frozen shoulders have a limited range of motion with their arms. By moving the place where the diaphragm inserts in the sternum (breastbone) this range can be increased. Every arm movement opens or loosens the chest, which is why we use arm movements so extensively. Arm movements supply oxygen, the fuel of energy, for all movement. Being out of breath is nothing else but becoming short of oxygen. The more space the body has for oxygen, for the air to come into the body, the more we have to move with. That is why it is important before doing anything else to do exercises that move the diaphragm and facilitate the intake of breath.

The heart supplies the right amount of oxygen needed for any given movement. When there is little oxygen coming into the body, the heart must work very hard to distribute it. When there is sufficient oxygen in the lungs for all the movements, the heart does not have to move as fast or as hard. By opening the chest and letting the air (breath) come in, the work of the heart is greatly facilitated. The heart is not strained when there is enough air entering the chest.

The chest can't stay open without correct support from the lower body. Therefore, correct positioning of the pelvis is very important. The pelvis can move along with the legs, if not held, and at the same time it can support the upper part of the body.

As the veins are worked both by the muscles and by the diaphragm, circulation is increased. Both diaphragm and musculature work against gravity to bring the blood back to the heart.

Releasing the Diaphragm

The diaphragm is the only muscle able to function in three dimensions. It moves from top to bottom, between front and back and all around the rib cage.

The way people breathe gives cues to whether or not they give themselves space to expand. The way one holds the body is a reflection of one's emotional life. We have different ways of holding ourselves protectively. We pull in, push down, or hold back, using our muscles.

One of the most interesting things about the diaphragm is that it is a connection between the involuntary and voluntary nervous system. It is thus a bridge between the unconscious and the conscious. As an interface between the emotions and the external world, the diaphragm is the ideal organ to work with and to observe. It is a barometer for one's being which reflects what is going on with a person. In the diaphragm, more than anywhere else in the body, we express emotional fluctuation.

Diaphragmatic movement is also important to circulation. Through the mechanics of breathing, the functioning of the diaphragm influences all the body's working organs. It is also the organ that makes it possible for us to have more oxygen in the chest with every breath.

To achieve a totally full breath, one must arrive at the point of releasing the diaphragm, which seems to be one of the most difficult things for us to allow. By putting a hand on the diaphragm area we teach people to become aware of how they control themselves. When people give up holding a position, the breath naturally enters the body. Infants can do it, animals can do it, but it seems to be an extremely difficult task for those of us who live in the modern world to let the diaphragm fully relax. When the diaphragm achieves full relaxation, the whole body works at its best.

Muscle Lengthening

A muscle has only two functions: to contract and to release. In order to move we must be able to relax. In order to have full motion one must be able to give up any kind of holding already in the muscle.

While movement of the joints is primary, opening and widening the chest is of equal importance. With the joints greased and the chest expanded, any kind of movement is possible.

Stretching, bouncing and swinging movements allow the muscle fibers to lengthen and loosen. The Rosen exercise routine is a logical means for allowing the body to move, and to move with ease. Moving with ease means eliminating all barriers we erect against movement. When the muscle is tense and it cannot contract, it cannot execute the movement. Strength is the possibility that exists between a muscle at rest and a muscle being fully active. We need to put the body in a position of non-doing so that strength and ability is available at any given moment to carry out any action.

When the muscles contract, there is less space than when the muscles are loose. It is basic to growth that one must give up the contracted space in which one corners oneself in order to find out how you are meant to be. Once we fill the space we were meant to fill, we seem to function fully, both on a physical and an emotional basis.

Tension is defined as nothing else but a muscle that has contracted and forgotten to let go. Life is a continual cycle of contracting and letting go. When you want to put out work, you contract; you go from not doing anything to a full contraction. When a muscle is tense, it is already contracted, and cannot do anything more because it has already been working. For the muscle to do work it must first be released. In Rosen's words, "It is really a place of non-doing that you start out with in order to do, in order to make use of your power. Relaxation prepares the body; makes the body ready and able to go into a state of doing."

Relaxation

Tension is holding muscles unconsciously in contraction. An enormous amount of energy goes into this. Vital energy that should be free for creative acts is directed into maintaining this contraction, although we are often unaware of this. The end result is the creation of a state where one is unable to begin movement fresh, from a relaxed state. *Holding is a barrier.* While tension is often required when moving, if tension is held when it is not required, it becomes an obstacle to the desired movement. Tightening also uses up a great deal of energy, so we are tired without having done very much real activity. Thus we need to use twice as much energy to accomplish our goals. Physically, great changes take place when we give up holding tension.

The tension we hold in our bodies is not life-promoting. Our power is available to us when we are undefended. Then we are free to move. That freedom gives us even greater power.

Reshaping the Body

Exercise creates a "conscious" body that can move everywhere, shaping itself according to the Greek ideal of beauty. It has the possibility of movement and good alignment. One of the most beneficial results for students working in Rosen Movement is the development of neuromuscular awareness. Once that consciousness is achieved, students leave class with a different attitude toward life. This awareness is psychological, physical, and emotional. It clarifies the self-image. A natural outcome for participants is that overall activity increases and illness is decreased. The awareness developed as a result of the exercises lasts longest if students participate weekly.

Feeling healthy is one of the most important basic conditions for an active life. When you do not feel good, it is difficult to feel a sense of enthusiasm for life. If we prohibit ourselves from living fully our body reflects our lack of enthusiasm.

Preparation of the Body for More Strenuous Movement

We want people to feel all the different possibilities they have in their bodies. We are eager for students to learn to be aware that the movements they do all day every day, like walking back and forth, are movements that count. Ideally Rosen work seeks to allow people to move fully, with joy and ease. These movements rearrange alignment and increase the body's capacity for action.

Rosen Movement is a learning/awareness process that allows people to feel movements on the inside that show on the outside. At the end of each class people feel energized and ready to dance.

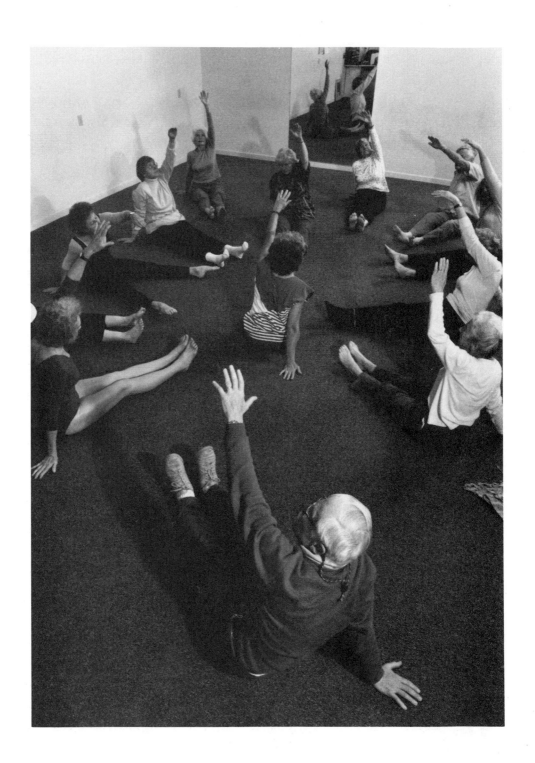

Chapter 2

The Class

People wear comfortable, loose, casual clothes: leotards and tights, or slacks and a tee-shirt. The room should be big enough so class members have enough space to move freely. Usually a classroom, gymnasium or dance studio is best, with the floor preferably carpeted for floor work. The classes are 50–60 minutes long and taught weekly. Temperature in the room should be comfortable; it should be well ventilated. Keeping consistent day and time are important. We begin with shoulder and chest exercises to provide necessary breath for the movements. Then we go into stretches so the muscles have their full length and are able to contract fully. Next we go to circle movements, mostly for the lower part of the body, to loosen up hip joints, and go through all possibilities the leg and foot can do. Thus prepared, we start to move more, using stepping, swinging of arms, turns. We are now ready to move across the floor where we combine the simple basic movements into dance like routines. We do this as long as class members have energy. These simple movements are fun, with lots of variations. Then we lie down on the floor, observe the breath, and begin movement directed to full flexibility of the spine. Also on the floor we have partner work. It seems we can take movements further when we work with a partner. We lie on our back, front, and side. We do slow and fast movements. The slow ones are designed to help us take inventory of our inner state through motion and breath. The faster movements are fun and give you a feeling of accomplishment. It is important at the end to have movement that is very satisfying so people leave feeling centered and joyful.

Warm-up

The purpose of the warm-up in the first part of the class, is to supply the oxygen necessary to do the movements that follow in more active parts of the class. Pectoral and shoulder movements open the chest. Rosen movement classes begin with upper body movements, stretching arms and shoulders which connect to the chest. With the chest open one can sustain movements without getting tired or out of breath. Therein lies the secret of why people in their seventies and eighties can still move vigorously—they have the oxygen they need for movement. When they stretch and move, there is no resistance. Their heart rates level off more quickly after vigorous exercise. People who come late for class and miss the warm-up do not get the benefit of the exercises. Their bodies do not change, and their tolerance toward exerting themselves does not change. So the warm-up is crucial. They should not miss it.

Circle

In the circle we begin to move the legs and hips in all directions in locomotion. We focus the work around the hip joint especially, which includes the relationship between leg and pelvis. By holding hands we make contact with others, and realize the physical support and stability others provide to move with ease. It is much easier to move when you are supported. The circle is a transition from the warm-up and preparation for later dancing across the floor movement.

Across the Floor

The second part of the class involves the entire body, now warmed-up. Students become aware of what they can do and take this possibility into more complicated sequences. Several movements are combined, and different movements are performed with different rhythms,

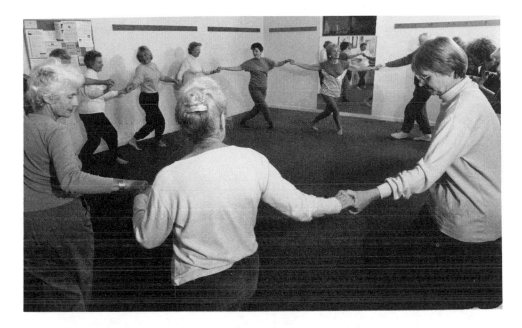

e.g., in waltz time, the fox trot, or a tango. People experience really dancing, performing the movements with abandon and joy rather than simply as exercise. They begin to move freely, to bring their own creativity to the movement.

All of the movements done prior to this stage prepare students for doing an across-the-floor segment with ease. Though it is a very effortless part of the class, it requires the most energy because more energetic movements are required. These movements would have been impossible to perform at the beginning of the class. Newcomers to the class think these tasks are impossible, but after they have done it for a while they find there's nothing to it. Very often they can do the exercises in correct alignment because the body has already learned how to do these movements. Students enjoy moving and take this ease and joy into their lives. We joke, but it is really true that we want our students to use these movements in their housework, in any kind of work they do. Every movement can be enjoyable, every movement can be a dance. To use movement as a dance, to dance through life—that is really our goal.

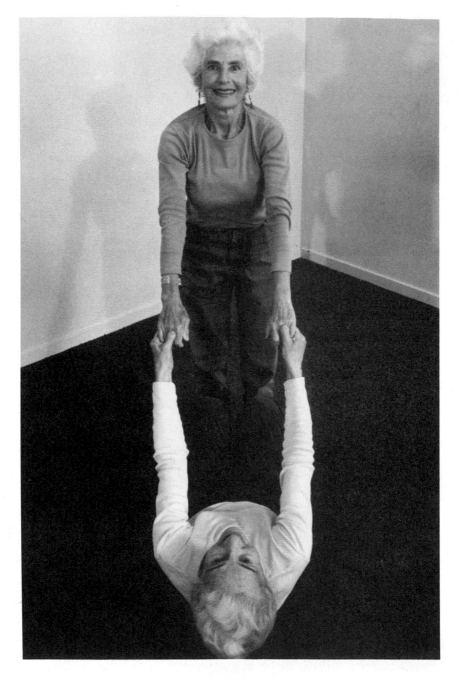

The See-saw (see p. 56)

Partners

The purpose of working with partners is to learn to adjust to each other in movement. Moving signifies being able to adjust to a partner or have a partner adjust to you in different ways. Partner work is used to teach techniques used in relationship. When classmates change partners and become acquainted with other people in the class, they learn to adjust to people. In the partner work students are asked to go a little further than they would go by themselves. The goal is to stimulate them to go as far as they possibly can in the movement with each other. Students are able to sustain exercises in partnership much longer than they can alone. It is encouraging and more fun than individual work.

Partner work creates safety, intimacy, a trusting relationship where people can work together with someone who can handle their body in a conscious way.

On the Floor

The floor movements are especially effective for the small musculature of the spine because they give the feeling of how the spine works as a whole. An example: when the knees are up and then fall to one side while the head falls to the other side, this stretch extends all the way through the spine. One can feel a slight torsion in every vertebra, one after the other.

There is always some tension in these little muscles when they have to hold the body in a standing position. When the body is lying on the floor, those muscles do not have to hold, and movement is fullest in this relaxed position. The muscles can relax, allowing for better results than when exercises are performed while standing. In the standing position there is room for one to compensate. But on the floor it shows what is and what is not within one's physical capacity. There is space to go a level deeper into the small musculature on the floor.

Floor exercises start with the big muscles, the outside muscles, so that they do not hold and immobilize us. By the end of the class these big muscles are moving with ease. It is very difficult to let the diaphragm relax fully when seated or standing. It is much easier to just let it go while lying down.

When students lie down on the floor, they are told to give up trying and let the abdomen fall towards the back. They know they don't have to hold up; they can trust the floor to hold them. The chest can also rest, and the diaphragm can swing.

Very often students are directed to lie on the floor after running around, having used their breathing possibility quite a bit. To level off when they lie down, they let the chest widen as much as possible. With every breath they bring a lot of oxygen into their system. The rapidity with which they level off indicates how relaxed they are. People who have been in the classes for a long time have no difficulty leveling off, but even young people, when they're new to the class, get out of breath because they cannot allow their chest to expand.

After the basic movements with the spine, exercises follow for the appendages: head, arms and legs, and through the small and big musculature of the back. These movements cover all the ways the vertebrae can move. Arm movements performed on the floor are very effective in stretching the chest.

The Plow involves coming up with the seat and taking the legs back behind the head. The Plow is a measure of how much the back and middle sections can be stretched. If students are relaxed, the feet can reach behind the head without any effort. This cannot be forced because it can cause pain if pushed, but done in a relaxed way it is a safe exercise for stretching the muscles along the spine.

When the little muscles are relaxed, the inner spaces in the spine become normal rather than too closely compressed. In the normal state they function towards one another, and it is in this movement that the synovial fluid, what keeps the joint functioning, can be created. One of Marion Rosen's discoveries in administering physical therapy was that shoulder pain occurred because people did not carry out movement fully. The part that was not moved was the source of pain. When one does not move, the joints cannot be lubricated. Relaxing the spine gives the small joints between the vertebrae the possibility for movement. The joint must be moved to its fullest during each class session to receive maximum benefit.

Focusing Attention in Teaching

In general, when teaching a group, it is important that you make some kind of a statement at the beginning, either with your body, your voice or with a gesture, letting people know that "Now I'm starting." With that movement or with what you say, you take responsibility for teaching the class. The knowledge that you are the teacher must come from you. That does not mean you have to be strict or strong. You have to be all there, present. You can use a soft voice, or a loud voice, but something must come through to the students that now you are starting a class. People who demonstrate authority teach a good class.

"I let my students talk in the class, and they can giggle," Marion Rosen has said, "but they have to do the exercises right. If they talk and do not pay attention to the exercises, then I say, 'You'd better watch. If they talk and do the exercises well, they can talk, because the talking and the expressing also have their place." We do not allow them to talk louder than we do, however, because it is important that our voices be the prominent one, the one to be heard. You can use your voice to explain as you go along what the movement is like and how you do it. Actually we all talk almost the whole time, to the group, while we move, while the music plays, while the other people talk to each other. When you want somebody to relax, of course you use a softer voice. If you want somebody to stretch, you stretch out the pronunciation. You cannot stretch with an abrupt command. The voice should match the movement.

There are several parts to the teaching. You should know how to develop your program, how to go through the body and what you have in mind to do. Secondly you should pick good music. Finally you should observe people carefully and really notice what they are doing. The tempo should always include the slowest person in class. Then you can speed up, but be sure that they all catch up with what you are doing. It is no fun to do it quickly with two or three people when the others are left behind, because when confusion occurs in one place, it seeps into the rest of the class. So there cannot be confusion. Sometimes students kick the wrong leg, or they do not quite know what to do, and you slow down a little bit so that they can catch up.

You also should be aware of when they get bored so that you can do something else. Even if you have prepared a wonderful program, let it go. If the students get tired, you cannot carry through a program. Be willing to let it go right in the middle of it. You can pick it up in another lesson, another class, and say, "Last time we did . . ." and then go a bit faster over what you prepared the previous time, and then you can do what you had planned to do in the first place. If they are too tired again, let go again. It is unnecessary to insist. If you plan correctly, very often you can go through to what you had planned to do. Always have something that will also get to the point where it will be fun for them.

It is important to take your cue from students rather than following a preconceived program. There should be no program, only people, and they should go home having received something. The most important part of the Rosen philosophy is that every class should have an impact on the people who attend. They should go home looking and feeling better.

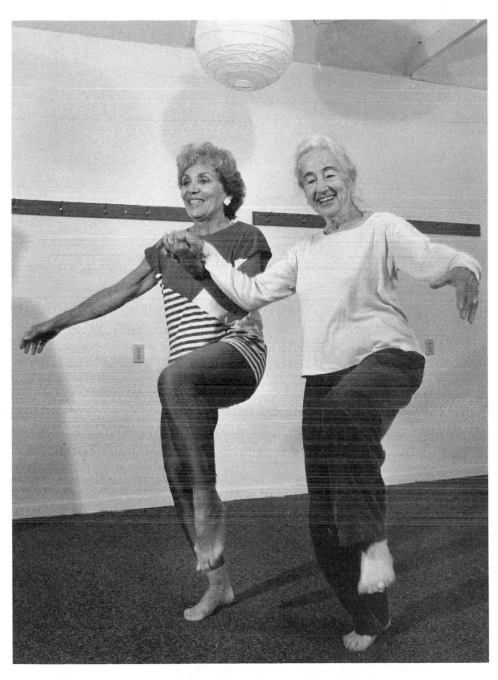

Frolicking at the ages of sixty-five and eighty-one.

Disabilities

Usually in a class there are quite a few people who have disabilities of some kind. The most common are sciatica, heart condition, light-headedness/dizziness, low back pain, and stiff necks.

Sciatica

Any movements between hips and legs are good for sciatica. Actually, whatever we do could not hurt a sciatica, but we are very careful when people bend over from the hip. We make sure movements involve only the hip joint and do not involve any bending higher up in the body, which is what causes a lot of their troubles. This stretches the hamstrings and muscles of the back and avoids pressure on the 4th and 5th lumbar vertebrae where the sciatic nerve emerges from the spine.

Bending and moving the hip joint is one of the most important things to help people with sciatica. Whenever there is pain, it is crucial to loosen up the muscle defense of the area involved. Very often the muscle defense causes more trouble than the condition itself. We clearly address muscle defense by loosening the secondary holding that accompanies pain. In the case of sciatica, attention is directed to the iliopsoas, the diaphragm, and the thigh muscles. The iliopsoas is a muscle located between the breastbone and the femur, whose action brings the vertebrae closer together. This often causes pressure on the emerging nerve. Another even more important consideration for sciatica sufferers is to learn to move with ease and to grasp the concept that movement does not require effort. Whenever we work with sciatica patients, we begin with the easiest letting go movements and end by "pushing a little bit."

The purpose of Rosen Movement is to create action, and to allow students to realize that this action can be done with ease. Rosen's philosophy is that if students have the ease to do a movement, they can repeat it, do it faster, and then do it in a way that does not hurt.

People with sciatica can also do abdominal floor exercises or sitting up exercises, which take strength, and force. These are the kinds of movements sciatica patients think they are unable to do. Any floor exercises, using one leg at a time, will loosen up the area around the hip, back connections and hip-leg connections. All are helpful for sciatica patients.

Leg lifts, one leg at a time (but never both together), are also helpful. It is important to do only enough movement to stay below the pain threshold and to go no further. If a person is apprehensive, she or he should refrain from doing a movement. Doing it in fear will cause holding, and pain.

It is very important that instructors of the Method be especially aware of persons in their classes with a tendency to sciatica and observe them to be certain they do not do anything to hurt themselves.

It is also important for instructors to backtrack again and again, to expand their peripheral vision, and be aware of everyone in the class. That is a good reason for keeping classes small rather than holding huge classes in big gymnasiums.

Heart Condition

Heart patients should always have a doctor's OK to participate in the class. Most of the Rosen movements are safe for heart patients, except those that involve jumping or very fast movements. With fast movements it is wise for instructors to watch for color in the face and how fast the students' breathing levels off.

"When I have somebody with heart trouble," says Rosen, "I do not do fast movements right away. I do a few fast movements the first time, and then have the person lie down. I watch how hard the breathing is, how long it takes to level off. Then I work with the letting go, especially when the person lies down. I want to show the person that there's a way to give space in their chest, for the air to come in."

Lying down on the floor, they are asked to let go of the chest and abdomen, which allows the air to come in and loosens the area around the heart. As the oxygen is replenished, the heart does not have to work so hard. When we hold, and don't let much air in, the heart has to work hard to make up for it.

Dizziness

Dizziness is caused by too much oxygen, and not enough oxygen in the brain. People get dizzy because they either don't breath enough, or are taking in too much breath. The neck muscles determine the right amount of oxygen. If they are tight, the exchange of oxygen to the head is impaired. When oxygen is allowed into the body, there is enough to distribute it with every breath.

When the movements are done correctly and the breath is allowed to come in, the eyes get very shiny, because this is one of the places where circulation is seen. The exchange of air between the head and the rest of the body must be open, or one will become dizzy. If dizziness or tetany occurs, contract, walk, move briskly throughout the room, and very soon there will be a leveling off of the breath and the conditions will disappear.

Lower Back Pain

Recurrent back pain may be the most debilitating of all disabilities because when the back hurts, there is pain no matter what position the body is in. Back pain is also very deceiving because the place where it hurts is usually not the source of the problem. The place where pain is felt is an effect of muscular contraction elsewhere.

Often people injure their backs in accidents. The place where the accident occurred often heals, but the position of holding adopted in response to the pain caused by the accident continues. Very often lower back pain is a manifestation not of the condition, or the injury itself, but of the aftermath, the habit pattern that developed after the injury. Rosen Method does not address the injury, but the attitude; the holding that occurs after injury. Healing is a general loosening up, a revitalizing of all the areas that have not been allowed to move. Holding a position is frequently quite painful for the back. The diaphragm may be held, or the back may be hyperextended to keep the injured area from hurting, but creating instead a very painful secondary situation. Our movements loosen up the areas that cause the condition. The diaphragm area is loosened by bending, stretching, by shoulder and torso movements, gently swinging, rolling, and by leg movements to loosen the lower part of the body. The Rosen Method works with the leg's connection to the hip and the way the legs are held.

The iliopsoas muscle, second only in importance to the diaphragm, should be loosened and stretched too. It serves as the important connection between the chest, the pelvis, and the legs, and works in connection with the diaphragm. The iliopsosas is located between the pelvis and the leg where the vena cava (the big vein that brings blood to the heart) runs from the leg into the body. If the iliopsoas and the joint between the pelvis and leg are tight, there will be pressure on the vein to the heart. As the vein already struggles against gravity to get the blood to the heart, one way to ease the function of the blood flow to the heart and to ease its transportation is by keeping that muscle working, rather than holding.

The small muscles at the bottom of the pelvis that rotate the legs in and out must move. Otherwise they stabilize the hip. It is necessary to destabilize movements so the muscles can be used again. If muscles don't give, if they are being held in some way, adjustment cannot take place. Even if only small muscles hold, the gross movements, like taking steps, cannot occur. Whenever muscles hold back, there is resistance, which causes discomfort and pain.

Most of the movements involving the back are either stepping movements or movements on the floor done with the legs. Because the lower back is particularly poorly constructed at the lumbar 4 and 5 levels, that area must be protected during the exercises. We avoid over-extending the back.

The fear of pain causes immobilization which in itself causes many of the actual dysfunctions of the body. Like joints getting stiff, muscles contract too much, creating poor circulation and poor oxygen supply. We can help reverse these conditions by slowly and gently helping people to start moving again. Movement *is* rehabilitation.

Stiff Neck

The neck is not just a "thing" stuck above the shoulders. The neck is the connecting link between the trunk and the head. The musculature connects the skull to the spine, the skull to the first and second rib and the clavicle between the top vertebra and the shoulder blade *(levator scapula)*. The muscles that move the neck reach to the chest area. Therefore, it is not enough merely to move the head or the neck. Movements designed for the chest are also very effective for the neck. Exercises for the muscles connecting the neck to the entire shoulder girdle, where they are attached and where they work from, are important. Whatever movements involve the shoulder girdle also influence the neck, as do any movements done in the top part of the thorasic spine.

After movements involving these areas have loosened up and the entire cervical spine has been limbered up, then the upper neck and head can move freely. Some of the muscles regulating the neck (the *scaleni,* which sit on the side of the neck) actually suppress emotion, earning the name "sadness" or "anger" muscles. The hiding *(levator scapula)* muscles elevate the shoulder blades. When the *omohyoid* and other hyoids on top of the rib cage, extending from the hyoid bone out to the sides, are tight they keep us from expressing emotions. Because it is difficult to devise movements that address these muscles exclusively, exercises that incorporate them into smaller movements of the shoulders and the upper chest are effective.

Pain

If a muscle has been held in contraction for a long time, that muscle is pretty sore when it does finally relax. This brings awareness of the strain that you have put on the muscle. A complete physiological change occurs in the area that was being held. When the blood first flows through that area, it hurts. There is an awareness of all the stiffness of an unmoving part. It is common that when someone is first loosened up, they become physically sore and experience pain. The instructor has not caused the pain; it has occurred because when one allows oneself to move, pain often is a temporary consequence.

Pain is caused through pressure on a nerve or by a constant pull of the muscle in the area in which it inserts. The muscle itself will hurt from having worked without rest. People come with chronic pain which physicians have had no way to deal with except medication. These conditions lend themselves very well to Rosen Method.

Sedentary and Stationary Work Styles

People who sit at desks or stand in one spot all day at their jobs establish an attitude, a way of being. Attitude is countered through movement. In the sitting position, the iliopsoas shortens and back muscles must hold in one position. Exercises that stretch the iliopsoas back and forth with hip movements, tilting the pelvis back and forth, help those who stand for long periods of time.

The pelvic rock is *the* most important exercise for sedentary individuals. Prolonged sitting very often affects the upper part of the back as well. Because sitting also demands upright posturing to balance, it is imperative to loosen the shoulder/chest area too.

For those required to do prolonged standing, hips, feet, and gross motor movements involving the legs (like stepping) are important.

Very often the feet are planted in one position. Movements that include bouncing, catching the weight, and pushing the weight up help the feet to stay flexible.

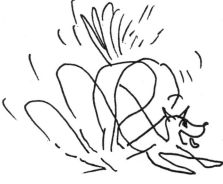

Preparing and greasing all joints for movement.
Wiggling all over, you provide your own physical therapy!

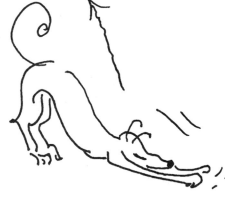

All the movements begin with a good s-t-r-e-t-c-h-!
To prepare yourself for movement, the muscles come to their full length and then are able to contract fully, making available the greatest potential for strength.

Chapter 3

Exercises

The exercises are designated for particular parts of the body. Coming from anatomic and kinesiological knowledge every exercise is given to produce a specific result. In order for the exercises not to be boring we have varied them in many ways. How this is done is up to the particular movement teacher. We have many exercises to choose from and can only do a few of each in every class. A teacher's skill shows in her or his ability to choose specific movements that meet the individual needs of students in the class. For this part of the book we have arranged the exercises in a workable class order. We begin with the chest because it contains the most significant organs—the heart and lungs. The lungs let the air in and the heart distributes the oxygen necessary for our bodies to move.

Shoulder Jog

Description: Bend your arms by the sides of your body. Move your elbows forward and backward, as a jogger does when running. Be aware of moving not only the shoulders and arms, but the center of the chest and the muscles that go from the shoulders to the neck.

Anatomy: Moves the whole upper part of the chest and the neck muscles, loosening up the shoulders, forward and back. The placement of the shoulder blades against the ribs is vital. All attachments between the shoulder blade and chest are being moved and result in chest expansion and a more freely swinging diaphragm.

Benefits: Moving the shoulder blades allows them to position freely. This gives the arm more strength, and is a basic movement we do with arms when we run. If we do this movement correctly, it enables us to jog with the least amount of effort.

Shoulder Jog

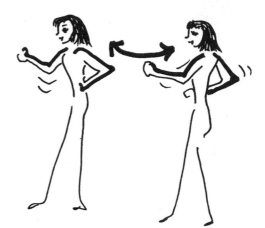

Wing Rock

Description: With bent arms rotated inward, alternately lift your elbows towards the ceiling. One should be aware of the loosening and opening of the rib cage, and the movement of the muscles between the head and shoulders.

Anatomy: By lifting the elbow you place the shoulder joint in position for maximum inward rotation. The bent arm position makes you move specifically in the shoulder joint. The back of the neck muscles (*levator scapulae, posterior scalenae*) are loosened as the transverse thorasic is moved.

Benefits: Shoulder joint movement keeps its range of motion. Without enough movement, it can become painful quickly.

Wing Rock

Hitch Hike

Description: Bend your elbow out to the side and in outward rotation. Lift the arms to shoulder height and backwards so the movement actually influences the shoulder and chest. Achieves the widest, most complete chest opening.

Anatomy: Works with the "lid" muscles (hyoid, *anterior scalenae*) to stretch the pectoral muscles. This creates movement in the muscles between the head and shoulders (trapezius), in the shoulder blades, and upper chest.

Benefits: Greases and frees the shoulder joint. Increases upper chest breathing capacity. The further you take the movement, the more the shoulder moves.

Hitch Hike

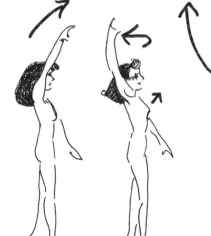

Stretch Up and Behind Ear

Description: Stretch your arm up above your head and move it back behind the ear.

Anatomy: Stretches the *latissimus dorsi* and pectorals.

Benefit: This movement keeps the joint from tightening up and gives the shoulder its full forward range.

Arm reaches back behind the ear.

Upper Chest Opening

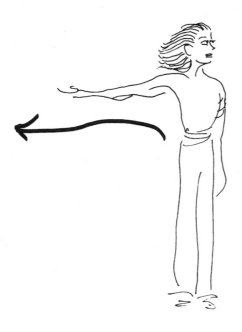

Description: Lift your arm forward on a horizontal plane, open out to the side and turn your head away in the opposite direction from the hand. Notice the stretch in the neck, chest and shoulder blade. Feel the room created in the upper chest.

Anatomy: Affects the neck muscles on the same side as the arm stretch. Stretches pectorals and opens the chest and transverse thorasic.

Benefits: Encourages full mobility between chest and neck.

We do not give head or neck exercises. We give shoulder exercises, and this is why. Most of the muscles that control the neck go to the shoulders, so whatever you do with the shoulders you do with the neck muscles.

You can allow the head to be free. You cannot *push* your head up. But you can allow yourself to pull down your shoulders and then let your neck lengthen. When the head comes out as far as you can allow it to, you then grow to your full height.

Opening Stretches for the Chest

Press Back

Description: With arms out to shoulder height, turn your palms forward and bounce your arms backward.

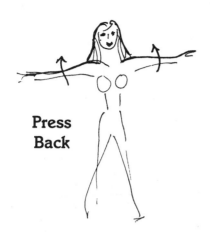

Press Back

Anatomy: Opens the chest and stretches pectorals and neck muscles attaching there. Stretches the deltoid.

Benefit: Opens the upper chest.

Rotation

Description: Arms out at shoulder height, one palm rotates forward and one backward. Alternate by turning hands.

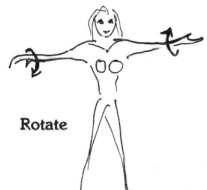

Rotate

Anatomy: Rotates *teres major* and minor muscles that come from the shoulder blade to the arm. Moves the "lid" muscles.

Benefits: Loosens up and greases the shoulder joint, reaches the transverse thorasic, deltoid, and pectoralis minor.

Embracing the World

Description: One arm straight forward, other arm straight backward with open chest. Turn torso to the side, palms up, lift sternum, look up and bounce arms backward. *Caution* Don't bend into lower back.

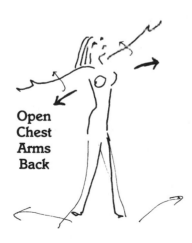

Open Chest Arms Back

Anatomy: Total opening of the chest, shoulder girdle and neck area.

Benefit: Stretches the diaphragm and gives the chest its greatest possibility of taking in air.

Open the Chest

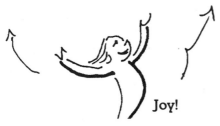

Gloom

**Concave
Hunch Over**

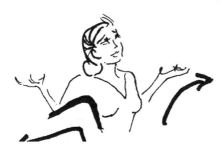

Joy!

**Convex
Open Out**

**Shoulders Back
Chest Open**

Description: To really loosen up the diaphragm, tilt it forward and backward at the level of the breastbone in front and twelfth thorasic vertebrae in back where the diaphragm is suspended. This movement makes us aware of the difference between depressed (slumping) position and a non-depressed (up lift) position.

Anatomy: Although a very small movement, it makes all the difference in the way the shoulder girdle adjusts itself and whether the diaphragm can really swing in the rest position.

Benefits: The amazing thing is that people can go through the exercise routines without being out of breath and without having to stop. The chest in the non-depressed position gives the possibility of moving, because with every movement done there is air coming into the chest.

Why don't people let the diaphragm move along with the rest of the body? The diaphragm is such a vulnerable area, and shows our emotions and our holding down and holding on. This is always the place where we do not give, we do not allow. You can really see the difference between depression and uplift when someone enters the room. You can see how someone feels when they walk in, depending on how they hold themselves in that area of their body. When the chest is up, then the arm movement and gestures you make are free and inviting.

Ribs

Description: Push ribs from side to side with hands on rib cage. Feel their mobility.

Anatomy: Enhances movement in the diaphragm and stimulates the breathing. Moves the muscular corset.

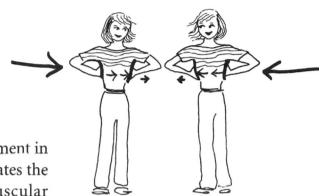

Ribs can move, side to side

Benefits: Increases breathing possibility.

Side Bend

Description: Lift one arm above your head and reach towards opposite side. Stretch and lengthen the same side of the body. To move there must be space between the vertebrae. If there is no space, there is no movement.

Anatomy: Stretches *latissimus dorsi*, oblique abdominals, *serratus* and small intercostal muscles.

Benefit: Flexibility of the rib cage.

A bit like an accordion.
Rib cage E-x-p-a-n-d-s on one side.
Rib cage Contracts on other side.

Stretch Up and Bend Over to One Side

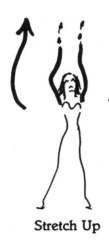

Stretch Up

Description: Lift both arms up to stretch as far as you can reach. From this position of length bend over at the hip joint and stretch one arm to the opposite side. Come up the same way, stretch in the middle, and go to the other side.

Anatomy: Stretches the trunk muscles in a slightly rotated position.

Benefit: Works all the trunk muscles and the *erector spinae* in a rotated position. Moves all the small musculature that rotate the spine.

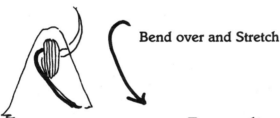

Bend over and Stretch

Accordion

Description: Reach out and stretch to one side. Extend the stretch by releasing the arm from the shoulder joint; take the head along. Move the arm sideways up and over the head towards the opposite side. Lengthening the trunk muscles, open up the rib cage. Stretch the small intercostal muscles (do *not* collapse to the other side) and lean slightly.

Anatomy: Releases muscles around shoulder joint. Muscular corset has to work lifting the chest up and over. Stretches trunk muscles and intercostal muscles.

Benefits: Mobility of the rib cage and all the muscles that cover it. Some mobility of the spine. Rib cage expansion allows breath expansion.

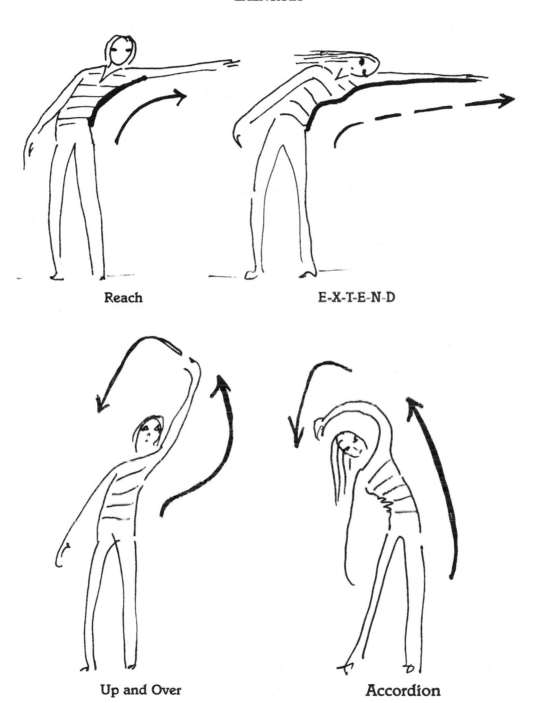

Reach

E-X-T-E-N-D

Up and Over

Accordion

Hang Loose

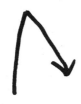

Description: With soft, unlocked knees bend at the hip joint. Rest belly towards thighs, let head go and dangle like a rag doll. Let the vertebrae have space between them. Come up slowly, unroll the spine vertebra by vertebra, pull up from seat muscles. Unroll lower, mid, upper back and finally head.

Anatomy: Lengthens *erector spinae* muscles that create space between the joints. Often relieves pressure on the invertebral discs. This allows for mobility of the spine.

Benefits: Hanging is relaxation and lengthens the muscles around the spine. More room in the joints for movement is created as the spine lengthens.

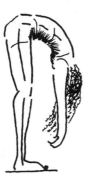

Bend Over

Windmill

Description: Hang forward, bending at the hip joint. Let the arms come backwards way up behind you. From that extreme position let one arm fall down while the other is still up; alternate. Move both arms backward, moving shoulder blade side to side. The higher the arms are in the back, the more satisfactory the movement.

Anatomy: Moves all the muscles that connect the trunk and shoulder blades. Loosens all the muscles that hold the shoulder blade in place.

Benefits: The correct position and adjustability of the shoulder blades in the back gives strength to the arm movements.

Windmill

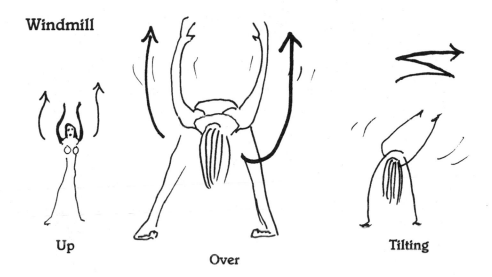

Up

Over

Tilting

Cleopatra

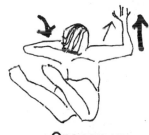

**One arm up,
one arm down**

Description: Bend your arms at shoulder height at right angles. Let one forearm go down and the other one up. Alternate a few times. Do this lying on your back or stomach. This is best done on the floor because the elbows are supported.

Anatomy: Moves the rhomboids, deltoid and trapezius as well as the upper thorasic and lower cervical spine. Moves the "lid" muscles.

Benefit: Moves the area around the dowager hump. It is the only movement we know that reaches this place specifically (see p. 79).

"Cleopatra"

Head Nodding (Saying Yes)

Yes

Description: Let the head fall forward; then bring it up with little effort. Let the top of the head lengthen towards the ceiling.

Anatomy: When you let the head fall forward all muscles that go from shoulders to the head get a passive stretch. Also the cervical part of the *erector spinae* is stretched. When we lift our heads up, shoulder, back, and head muscles contract (*levator scapula,* posterior *scalenes*).

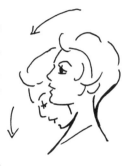

Benefit: Vertebrae of the cervical spine are moved towards each other so the joints get their necessary movement.

Say Yes

Head Side-to-Side

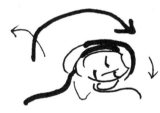
Head Side-to-Side

Description: Let the head fall to the side, lift it up easy and let it fall to the other side, looking forward. Allow movement to be felt in the chest.

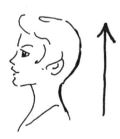

Anatomy: Stretches both *scalenae* and trapezius. Head moves but this is a neck muscle and cervical vertebrae movement.

Benefit: Increased movement in shoulder-neck connection. Sideways movement in joints of the vertebrae.

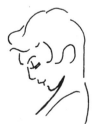
Say Yes

Hip Swings

Description: Let the hip come out to one side and put the weight on one leg with slightly bent knees. Alternate side to side; it becomes a wiggle.

Anatomy: Stretch the *tensor fascia lata* and *glutei.*

Benefit: More free hip movement.

Hip Swings

Hip Circles

Description: Circle the hips as far as they will go in all directions.

Anatomy: Involves all the muscles around the pelvic area.

Benefit: Moves the organs in the pelvic area. Stimulates blood flow and digestion.

Hip Circles

Step Forward

Description: Step forward and put weight on forward leg. Movement between hip, one leg, then the other, and upper torso.

Anatomy: Moves the sacroiliac and pelvis floor muscles. Loosens up muscles around the hip joint.

Benefits: Ease in movement of hip joint.

Step/Weight

Step Forward and Backward

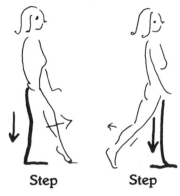

Step   **Step**

Description: Step forward and backward, with the weight on the supporting leg. Movement between hip and leg.

Anatomy: Moves and stretches the iliopsoas and *glutei*.

Benefit: Loosens up hip joint.

Swing Leg Forward

Description: Lift leg straight forward from hip joint.

Anatomy: Movement in hip joint, works hip flexors.

Benefit: Mobility of hip joint. Stretches hamstrings and strengthens flexors.

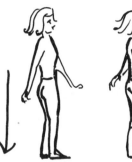
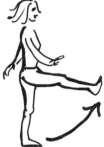

Swing Leg Forward

Back Scissors

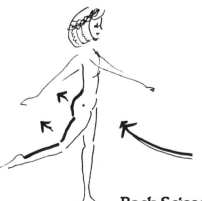

Back Scissors

Description: Swing leg backward at hip joint. Keep low back straight.

Anatomy: Mobilizes more of hip joint. Stretches iliopsoas, works *gluteus* muscles and hamstrings.

Benefit: More fun active movement.

Lift Lower Leg Back

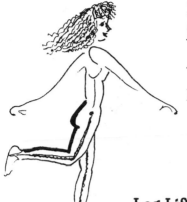

Description: Bend knee backward from the hip joint.

Anatomy: Stretches iliopsoas and chest.

Benefit: Stretches whole frontal side of body.

Leg Lift Back

Pelvic Rock

Description: Stand with one leg forward, one back. Lower your seat backwards over back leg bending hip joint, weight on back leg (like sitting on a stool). Shift weight of pelvis over the forward leg straightening out the hip joint, so your weight is directly over the pelvis.

Anatomy: Alternately relaxes and contracts the iliopsoas, gluteus, and hip joint.

Benefit: Puts pelvis in position to best support the rest of the body in walking. Allows possibilities of free movement in hip joints. Basic walking movement.

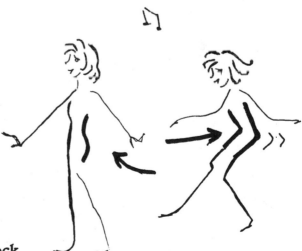

Pelvic Rock

Knee Twist

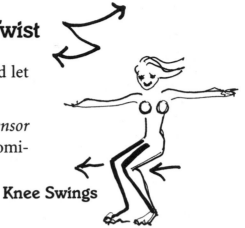

Description: Bend knees slightly and let them swing side to side.

Anatomy: Moves *gluteus* muscles, *tensor fascia lata* and iliopsoas, oblique abdominals.

Benefit: Mostly for fun.

Knee Swings

Toe and Heel Twists

Description: Rotate the hip joint inward and outward by pointing toes out and in as far as possible. Be sure to keep the hip joint facing forward.

Anatomy: All the muscles between the leg and pelvis are involved, including some of the deep pelvic muscles.

Benefits: Loosens up musculature around the hip joint. Stimulates deep pelvic muscles which hold the sexual organs and intestines.

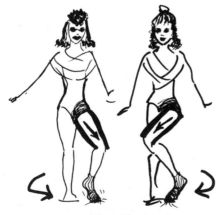

Toe Twists

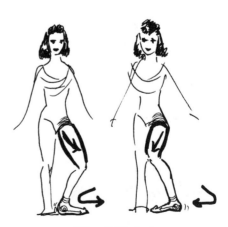

Heel Twists

Heel Lift

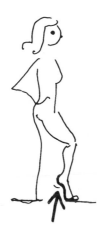

Description: Stand with your weight on one leg and lift the other heel with the toe on the ground.

Anatomy: Loosens small joints of the foot.

Benefits: Prepares the foot for movement.

Heel Lift

Grapevine

Description: Lift your leg and cross step in front and back alternately.

Anatomy: Enhances movement of muscles in the pelvis and also between the leg and pelvis. Movement of gluteus, hip flexors and extensors, and sacroiliac joint. At the same time creates counter movement in the upper trunk through the chest and shoulder area.

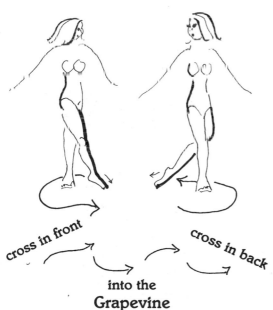

cross in front   cross in back

into the
Grapevine

Benefits: More breathing space. Connects chest and pelvic movements. Lots of fun!

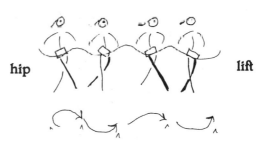

hip   lift

Whole group joins in a circle, doing the grapevine, a leg movement involving the upper body as well. This movement becomes a dance.

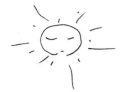

Rest

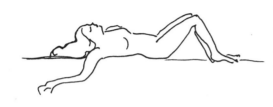

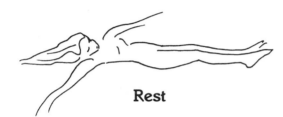

Rest

Description: Lying on your back, straighten out the legs or put feet on the floor with knees bent. Relax the abdomen towards the floor. Let the back rest totally on the floor. Let the chest expand and allow the breath to come in. Let the neck lengthen. The head should touch the floor without using any effort.

Anatomy: Awareness of non-doing. Lying without doing anything.

Benefits: Diaphragm can move freely. Abdomen can relax fully.

Pelvic Lift

Description: Lie on the floor with knees bent and feet touching the ground. Relax thigh muscles, allowing motion in the hip joint. Lift the seat, pushing with hips upwards (not abdomen) to lift. As you let yourself down, relax hips and lengthen spine vertebra by vertebra.

Anatomy: This movement is for the sacrum and all the back vertebrae so they will move back and forward towards each other.

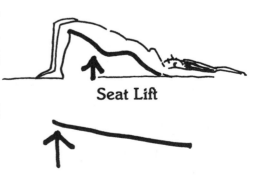

Seat Lift

Benefit: Provides mobility around the sacroiliac and hip joint.

Knee Flops

Description: Lie on back, knees bent, feet on the floor. Flop knees together to one side and at the same time turn head in the opposite direction. Alternate. The arms are out to the side horizontally, shoulder high.

Anatomy: Reaches erector spine complex, from pelvis to head. Mobilizes the whole spine.

Benefits: Movement in knees. Action in hip joint and whole spine. Mobilizes the entire trunk area.

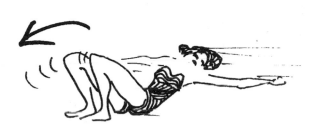

Knee Flops

Hamstring and Abdominal Series

1.

Description: Lie down, knees bent, feet on floor. Take one knee up to the chest and straighten it. Extend it toward the ceiling and bounce toward the nose. Bend and return to original position. Alternate.

Anatomy: Stretches ham strings and gluteus.

Benefit: Also stretches lower back.

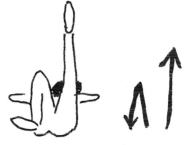

1. One leg extended.

2.

Description: Pull one knee up, then the other. Extend one leg and then the other toward ceiling. Bounce toward nose. Bend knees one at a time and return to original position.

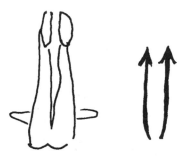

2. Both legs up.

Anatomy: Stretches lower back. Enhances mobility in the lumbar area.

Benefit: Disk problems can be avoided.

3.

Description: Pull one knee up to the chest and then the other. Circle knees three times in each direction. Return to original position.

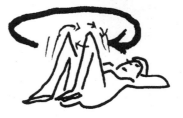

Anatomy: Works the abdominal muscles.

3. Knee circles.

Benefit: Increases support for the intestines and muscular corset.

4.

Description: Raise the knees to the chest and place hands on top of knees. Extend one leg and flex the other alternately. Motion brought about by hands, not legs, is felt in the chest and hip joint.

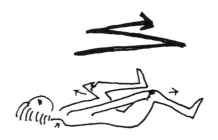

Anatomy: Stretches *gluteus* and lower back. Mobilizes neck and shoulders.

4. Cable car lying down.

Benefits: Increases movement in neck, shoulders and hip joint.

Side Leg Lift

Description: Roll to side, one hand in front, palm down to support body. Head rests on the arm of the same side. Lift both legs off floor simultaneously, keeping them touching together and parallel.

Anatomy: Involves all the abdominal muscles and the abdominal corset. This movement strengthens the stomach by engaging all these muscles. They hold in the intestines and support the contents of the abdominal area.

Benefits: Often used for people with back pain and after giving birth.

Side Leg Lift

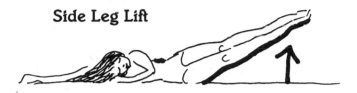

We say "Take your stomach along." Very often people are holding their stomachs out. As they move around they don't move their stomachs. Your stomach should move along when your hips move from side to side. Of course, it's very important that the stomach is relaxed because when you do any kind of a stretch when the stomach is pushed out, you don't get a stretch. You have to be aligned in order to get a good stretch.

Leg Circles

Description: Lie on your back and your lift legs one at a time toward the ceiling. Make a small circle and then bigger ones three times each direction with both legs.

Anatomy: Strengthens the oblique abdominals.

Benefit: Strengthens the muscular corset.

Leg Circles

Feet

The foot is a very important part of the body. It carries the weight and connects our beings to the ground. The foot has the most joints in a small area of the body. Every joint needs to be moveable towards its neighbors in order to be of greatest use to us. The foot carries our weight, bounces us forward and catches us when we jump. In locomotion the foot plays the biggest part. Standing in one place it influences the alignment of the whole body.

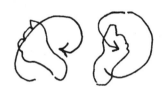

Ankle Circles

Description: Lie on your back, knees bent toward chest and circle ankles in both directions.

Anatomy: Outward rotation of hip. Works all the lower leg muscles.

Benefit: Loosens up muscles that tend to hold ankles stiff.

Ankle Circles

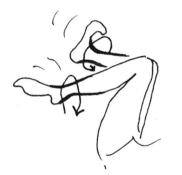

Foot Flops

Description: Lying on your back, legs apart, let both feet flop towards and away from each other. Movement in hip joint.

Anatomy: Leg rolls in hip joint.

Benefit: Greasing the hip joint.

Foot Flops   Toward, away

54

Foot Rolls

Description: Lie on back, feet parallel, legs straight on the floor. Flop both feet side to side. Movement in hip joint.

Anatomy: Leg rolls in the hip joint.

Benefit: Greasing the hip joint.   **Foot Rolls**

Knee Hug

Description: Bend both knees to the chest, hug them and rock forward and backward. The lower back is in a totally protected position; you can do all kinds of movement this way without hurting the lower back.

Anatomy: For the lower back.

Benefit: Rolling the vertebrae toward each other when you are rocking side to side reaches the sacroiliac and the hip joint. All the muscles around the hip joint are being gently moved.

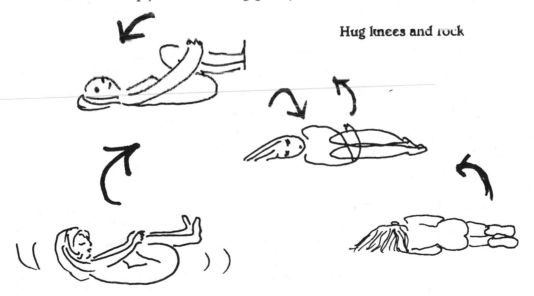

Hug knees and rock

See-saw

Description: One leg straight and the other bent, hands around one knee. You rock without effort because the weight of the straight leg takes you forward; your momentum brings you up again. The free leg works as a lever to bring you up as well. Alternate sides.

Anatomy: Moves the lower back. This is one of the best back exercises for loosening up.

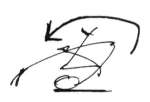

Rock up — Rock back
See-saw

Hug one knee.

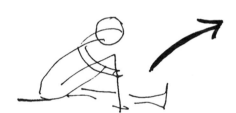
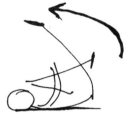

Sit Ups

Description: Sit up, reach hands towards feet and rock back and forth from the hip joint until your hands touch your toes.

Anatomy: Lengthens the lower back and stretches the hamstrings.

Benefit: These muscle areas are stimulated to their natural working capacity.

Sit Ups

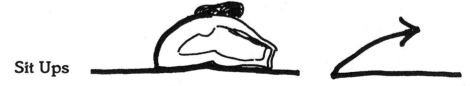

Shoulder Stand

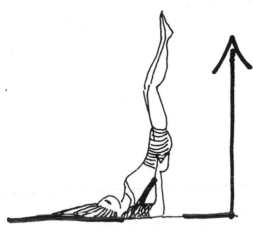

Description: Roll on your back, lift up your seat, and extend both legs towards the ceiling until your weight rests on your shoulders.

Anatomy: A strengthening exercise for the muscular corset.

Benefits: Stretches lower back. Strengthens the muscular corset, abdominals and *quadratus lumborum*.

Shoulder Stand

Foldover

Description: From the shoulder stand let one leg go behind your head on the floor and then the other leg so both touch the ground. You must relax your diaphragm to allow the bend to happen.

Anatomy: Stretches the entire *erector spinae*. Involves the big and small musculature because each vertebra is bent in order to achieve this. You must relax the diaphragm and abdominal muscles. When we reverse the movement to come up, we engage the muscular corset again. When we sit up afterwards, the legs are straight on the ground and the arms reach forward toward the toes. This affirms the stretch that has taken place because you can see how much further you can stretch than before.

Benefit: To stretch the whole spine; an easy passive stretch.

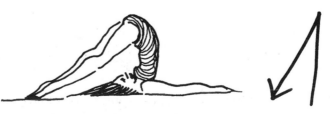

Foldover

Lower Leg Flop

Description: Lie on stomach, knees bent and head resting on hands. Let both lower legs flop side to side.

Anatomy: Stretches the hip rotators, especially the iliopsoas. This loosens up the mid back, the area of origin of iliopsoas.

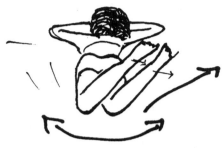

Windshield wipers

Benefits: This is an easy limbering up movement for the iliopsoas and both its attachments. Secondarily, the diaphragm is influenced.

Knee Lift

Description: Lie on the stomach, knees bent and head resting on hands. Lift and lower one leg at a time, alternating, toward ceiling.

Anatomy: A stretch for the abdominal muscles, iliopsoas, *rectus femoris*.

Benefits: Stretches and relaxes the flexor muscles of the hip.

Leg Lift

Description: Lie on the stomach, legs straight, head resting on hands. Lift legs alternately straight backwards.

Anatomy: Stretches flexors and makes extensors work.

Benefits: Stretches front of hip and strengthens extensors.

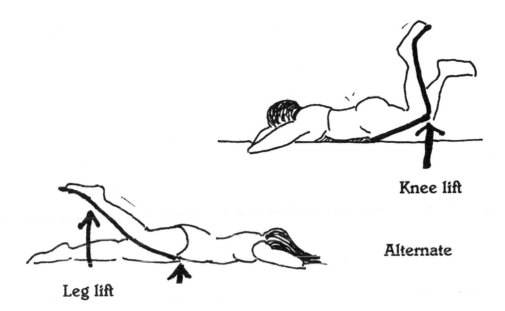

Knee lift

Alternate

Leg lift

Flop Heels

Description: Lie on the stomach, bend the legs up and rest head on hands. Flop legs apart and together.

Anatomy: Stretches adductors, and deep hip rotators.

Benefit: Releases adductor tension.

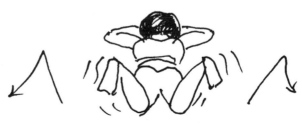

On stomach - flop heels

Chapter 4

Sequences

The purpose of a sequence is to create a series of movements to mobilize a particular part of the body. The student should fully use and integrate this moving part with other parts of the body. These sequences are done throughout the class. We choose from among the following sequences those that accomplish a certain objective. All of these movements enable and encourage people to retain mobility as they grow older. Our oldest pupil is presently eighty-three years old.

Opening The Chest

1. One partner sits while the other partner stands behind her with knees gently bent against the sitting partner's back, supporting her.

2. Standing partner: gently bounce your knees into your partner's back. Massage it by walking your knees up and down her back slowly.

3. Hold her hands. Move your arms out to the side with the elbows bent. With her arms

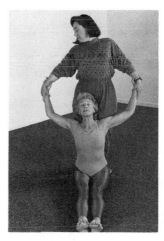

3.

held apart, turn her torso side to side in order to achieve movement and stretch in the chest.

4. In the same position, move her arms forward and backward, stretching her chest wider and wider.

5. With elbows bent and out to the side at shoulder level, pull up with one arm and stretch to lengthen the side of her body. Alternate with the other arm.

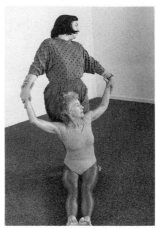

3.

6. Lower your arms.

7. Place both hands on her shoulders and push down gently.

8. With your hands still on her shoulders, pull gently back to open your partner's chest.

9. Push her forward all the way down from the shoulders and upper back, then bounce gently, and return to sitting. The bend is in the lower back and hip joint.

10. Standing in front of your partner, whose knees are bent, take both her hands and pull her up to standing.

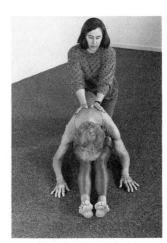

9.

11. Finally, reach up, hands and arms extending high into the air, into a big stretch.

12. Switch partner positions and repeat the entire sequence.

This sequence opens the upper part of the chest and stimulates the diaphragm, stretching pectorals and transverse thorasic.

Shoulder Joints and Chest: the Scarf

1. The instructor distributes one five- to six-foot-long scarf per student. During this sequence keep the scarf taut whenever possible.

2. Unfold the scarf as wide as you can. Holding both ends, lift it up above and a bit behind your head. Lower your arms. This movement gives a forward flexion of the shoulder joint.

3. Lift your arms above your head. Maintain a midline position and twist from the shoulders three times, rotating the shoulder blades. Then lower your arms.

4. Rest a moment.

5. Lift your arms up above your head and stretch them apart again. With your arms above your head, lean your body towards one side and then the other, repeating three times. Lower your arms. This stretches the connections between the waist, shoulder and pelvis.

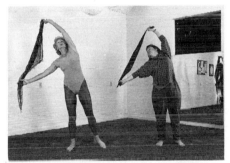

5.

6. With both hands holding the scarf, lift it in front of your body, arms apart. Lower your left arm down and raise the right arm up, alternating three times.

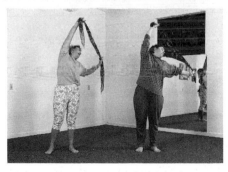

5.

7. Hold the scarf taut at both sides. Lift both arms to one side, turn your head and look under your arm. You should feel a stretch along your rib cage.

8. Face forward and continue the movement, circling overhead with one arm leading and the other following along with it.

9. With both arms in front and to the sides, lift the scarf up over your head and lower it down behind your body. Reverse direction and repeat slowly three times.

10. Lower your arms in front of you and step over the scarf. Take it up, behind, over, and down in front of your body. Repeat.

11. Move the scarf behind your body and lift it up as far as you can.

12. Add a bend in the hip joint, letting your arms come up as far as possible. Sway with both arms side to side.

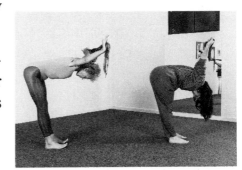

12.

13. Come up slowly to standing.

14. Rest a moment.

15. Hold the scarf in one hand and swing it in small circles, shoulder-high. First swing it from the wrist. Then, bending the elbow, make the circle bigger until, finally, it circles all the way around your body, overhead like a lasso.

It is more fun to stretch with an object. Students can choose which scarf they like. They can stretch a little further when the scarf is held in a certain plane. Whatever the teacher can do to bring out the class's active involvement helps enhance our students' enjoyment.

Head Stretches for the Neck

These movements are passive for the receiver or sitting partner. She should totally relax and allow her limbs to be moved by the standing partner.

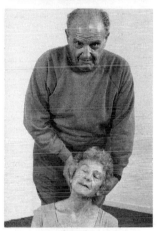

1.

1. One partner sits while the other stands behind her with his knees supporting her back.

2. Standing partner: with both hands, hold the sides of her head and rotate it gently.

3. Tilt her head slightly side to side.

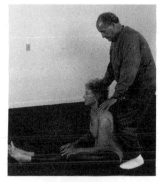

3.

4. Lift her head up and lower it a few times with your hands under the mastoid bone (behind the ear).

5. Keep one hand under the mastoid bone and move the other under her chin. Lift and lower her head a few times, slowly.

6. Placing your hands on the sides of her head, lift and turn it side to side. Return to center. Lift and turn to the other side, return to center, and rest. Repeat a few times very slowly.

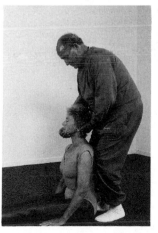
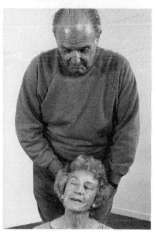

6.

5.

7. Tilt her head towards her shoulder, then return it to the center. Tip and tilt slowly on the other side. Repeat a few times.

8. Hold your partner's head with both hands and freely move it around in all directions.

9. Place one hand on the ocipital line (base of the skull) and the other hand on the forehead. Nod her head forward and backward.

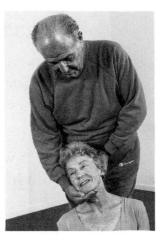

7.

10. Bend your knees into your partner's back and bounce slightly.

11. Continue bouncing, and with your hands on your partner's shoulders, pull them back.

12. Push her shoulders forward. Her head should relax. (The sitting partner can stretch her arms forward to touch her toes.)

13. Again with your hands on the ocipital line and chin, lift your sitting partner up tall. Then support her head as you lower your partner backwards to the floor. The passive sitting partner tries to relax like a rag doll, giving you her full weight.

14. Lie down next to your partner on the floor and breathe easily.

Free movement of the neck and shoulder area seems very important to a person's well-being. This sequence helps to clear the head for thinking and for looking in all directions.

Neck Sequence

People always complain of having stiff necks. We developed these routines to help them. These slow stretching movements reach many muscles that connect the neck to the rib cage and shoulder girdle.

1. Begin standing. Lift one arm overhead and move it back behind the ear. Repeat on the other side.

2. Adding a collapse in the chest, repeat the movement. Touch your sternum with your other hand and see how far your arm moves now. Repeat on the other side.

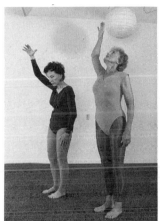

1.
2.
3.

3. Return to the uncollapsed position and pull your arm back as you did in step 1.

4. Touch your sternum with both hands. Lift your elbows up and down.

5. Move one elbow back as far as you can go; return to center. Move the other elbow back and return to center. Feel the movement through the shoulder girdle and upper chest.

6. In unison, move both elbows forward and backward.

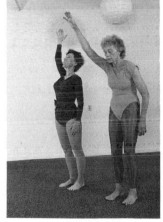

1.
2.
3.

7. With your hands on your collarbone, lift your shoulders up and let them drop. Feel the way your collarbone rides on your rib cage.

8. Placing your hands on your collarbone, lead with your elbow. Move the right shoulder forward and twist your upper torso towards the rear. Then bring the left shoulder forward to the center. Reverse

the movement. You will feel a stretch around the clavicle and shoulder girdle.

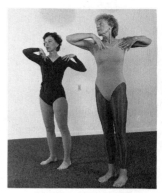

8.

9. Now raise your arm again behind your ear and see how much further you can take this stretch.

10. Touch your collarbone with your left hand and stretch your right arm out to the side and backwards.

11. Then turn your head to the opposite side of the extended arm as far as possible. This will stretch the entire shoulder-head connection. Repeat on the opposite side.

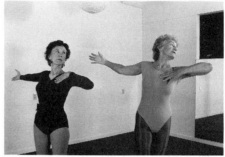

11.

12. Raise both arms up and behind your ears, then lower both arms by your sides and continue to move them backwards while you bend down at the hip joint. Pull your arms backward and up as far as you can.

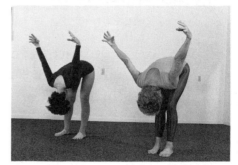

12.

13. Come back to a standing position.

14. When your arms are backward and up as far as possible, let one arm drop to the floor, keeping the other up behind you. Alternate three times.

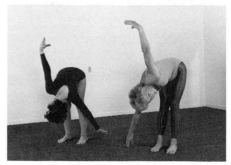

14.

15. Stand up again.

16. Reach behind you with your right arm and touch your left shoulder blade. Reach your left arm forward as far as you can and then retract the straight left arm as far as possible. Note with the right hand the movement of the shoulder blade. Alternate sides, noticing the action of your shoulder blades.

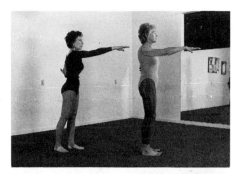

16.

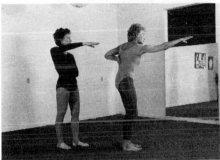

16.

17. Imagine your hands on a steering wheel. Turn your head side to side and see how far back you can look. Can you back out of your garage now?

All the movements we did in this routine lessen stress, pain and stiffness in the muscles that inhibit action of the head and neck. Completing this sequence will help you to regain better range of motion in these areas.

Shoulder and Neck

1. Stand facing each other with palms touching. Raise your arms in front to shoulder level, pushing one arm forward and pulling the other back. Alternate, moving with the music a few times.

2. Facing each other, turn your hands inwards, elbows to the outside. Then turn your hands outside and your elbows inside (windshield wipers). Repeat three times.

3. With your hands on each others' shoulders, push one shoulder forward, pulling the other gently back.

4. With your palms together, lift one elbow up and out to the side and look underneath through the opening three times. Then do the movement on the other side.

5. Arms down and holding hands, raise each of your arms, one side at a time, until you make an arch above your head and look through the opening. Repeat on the opposite side. (In class we call this Look Through the Window.)

6. Continue this movement, turning into the opening until your bodies have made a half circle and you are back to back. Pause, and let the chest be opened by this stretch while your hands are still clasped behind you.

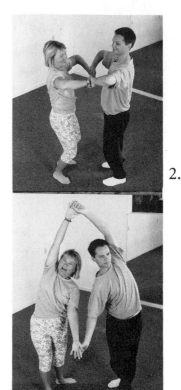

2.

5.

5.

7. Return to facing each other by reversing the movement. Repeat it on both sides two times, very gently.

8. Place both your palms together in the middle again. Lift your hands up the center of your bodies and circle wide, out to the side.

9. Reverse, moving up from the sides, over your heads, down to a middle line in front of you, moving down. Repeat three or four times.

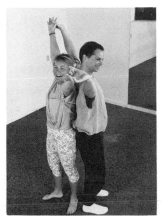

6.

10. With palms together, reach your right arms out to the right side. Lean your head to the right side, then return to the middle. Do the movement to the left side three times.

These sequences stretch the sides of the rib cage and the muscles that connect the back to the shoulder, as well as the *latissimus dorsi*.

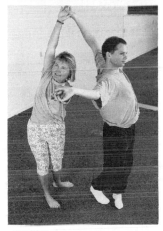

7.

Hips and Ribs: the Subway

1. Imagine that you are on a subway. Reach one arm upwards as far as you can, stretching towards an imaginary strap. Repeat two times with each arm.

2. Rest.

3. Return to holding the strap. Rock your hips from side to side. Alternate arms.

4. Hold on with the right hand and move your hips in a full circle to the right. Repeat, using the left hand, circling to the left.

5. Rest.

6. Holding the strap, alternately lift one hip at a time. (Your feet remain on the floor.)

7. Holding the strap, put one foot forward and the other back. Shift your weight forward and backward over the hip joint with your weight-bearing knee bent. Alternate arms and legs, and repeat.

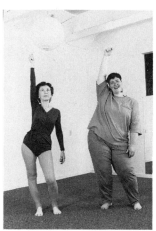

6.

8. Holding on to the strap with your legs side by side, bend your knees and rock forward and backward from the hip joint. Do the same movement double time.

This sequence stretches the muscular corset between the hips and rib cage, loosening the muscles around the hip joint and playing with weight and balance.

Chair

You can do this in a wheelchair, an airplane, seat, or anywhere you must remain seated for a long period of time.

Neck/Shoulder area:

1. Lift one shoulder up and down, then do the same movement on the other side.

2. Move one shoulder forward, the other backward, while maintaining a midline position.

3. Look slowly over one shoulder and then the other.

4. Lift and lower both shoulders.

5. Hitchhike: Look straight ahead, arm stretched out to the side at shoulder height. Turn your thumb out and back with your elbow bent. Alternate sides.

6. Hitchhike: Do the same exercise again, but look in the opposite direction of your thumb.

6.

7. Hands held loosely at your thighs, bend side to side with head and chest.

8. Bend to one side. Inhale when you come to the middle and breathe out as you bend to the other side.

9. Drop your head forward to lengthen the back of the neck.

10. Nod from where your head and neck come together (ocipital ridge).

11. Drop your head lower to lengthen the spine.

12. Rotate your head from side to side (first slowly, then faster).

Hip area:

13. While sitting, hold on to the seat of your chair. Lift one knee and put it down. Alternate with the other side three or four times.

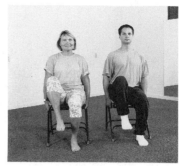

13.

14. Holding on to the seat of your chair, cross your legs at the knee. Alternate with the other leg three or four times.

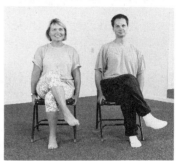

14.

15. Lean forward from the hip joint. Look side to side and reach out as if to pick something up from the floor.

16. Holding on to the arm rests, lift up one buttock, then the other.

17. Hold on to the arm rests and lift up your seat as high as possible; then sit down again, pushing off from the floor.

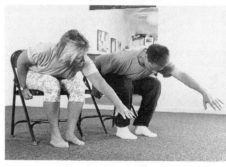

15.

18. Lean over and rock forward, lifting seat as if to leave the chair.

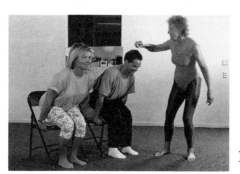

17.

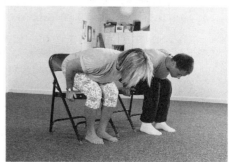

18.

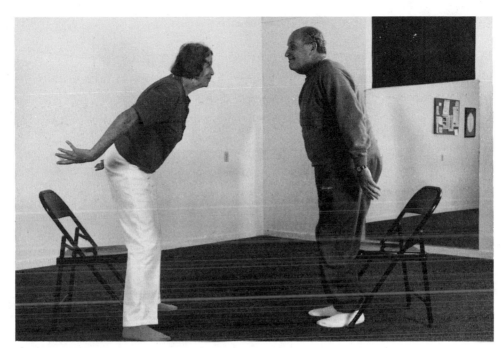

19.

19. Continue this motion until you are standing if you can.

Feet:

20. Roll both feet from side to side.

21. Tap one foot at a time, heels staying on the ground.

22. Lift toes, one foot, then the other.

23. Lift heels, one foot, then the other.

24. Point toes out to the side and then bring them back to the middle.

25. Move heels out to the side and back to the middle.

26. Move toes out and in, heels out and in.

27. Sway both knees side to side.

28. Pull both knees apart and then squeeze them together.

Face:

We have habitual expressions which freeze on our faces. We forget what else our faces can do or express. This exercise is to help make you aware of what you can show in your face.

29. Grin as wide as possible.

30. Dead pan (solemn, stern).

31. Blow (puff cheeks up).

32. Grin and blow, grin and blow.

33. Squeeze eyes.

34. Open eyes as wide as possible.

35. Wrinkle your nose and look down on somebody.

36. Stick your chin out forward and then pull it back as far as you can.

37. Frown.

38. Relax.

39. Look up, look down, frown, let go. Repeat.

40. Grin again.

41. Let your face be at rest, eyes open, no position held. Let yourself be seen the way you are.

Working with the Back

1. The position to be used for movements #2–8 is as follows: Lie on your back with knees bent, feet flat on the floor, weight through the feet, arms out to the side. Relax the thigh muscles.

2. Begin by lifting your lower back and seat up from the floor. Then lower slowly, relaxing, vertebra by vertebra. This moves the whole spine. Be sure to relax totally before you raise up again. You do not need to contract the buttocks. The movement comes from the hips and erector spinae muscles.

3. Raise one knee to the chest and lower, then the other. Alternate four times.

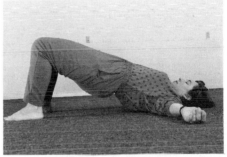

2.

4. Straighten one leg at a time up toward the ceiling with the flat of the foot parallel to it. Then lower, returning to bent knee position. Alternate. This movement stretches the hamstrings.

5. Straighten one leg towards the ceiling and bounce it toward your nose gently. After lowering the leg, take time to breathe and relax the abdomen. Alternate.

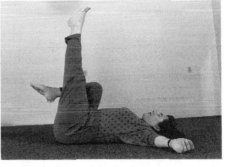

4.

6. Bring both legs up, one at a time, and bounce them both gently towards your nose. Bend your knees before bringing the legs down in order to protect the lower back, and then lower them to the floor.

7. Let your feet rest on the floor and relax the thigh muscles. Let both knees fall to the right side. Return to the middle with little effort,

then let both knees fall to the left. Alternate a few times.

8. Let both knees fall to the right side, turning head to the left. Then let both knees fall to the left side, turning head to the right. Continue alternating sides a few times, slowly feeling the movement through the entire spine.

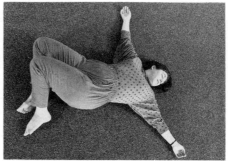

8.

9. Roll to the right side. Stretch your right arm above your head and place your head on it, putting your left hand flat in front of you on the floor for support.

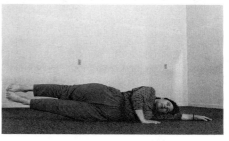

9.

Make sure you are totally in a straight line, upper leg on top of lower leg. Lift both legs together at a 35–45 degree angle from the floor a few times. This strengthens the muscular corset and whole trunk.

10. Extend one leg forward as far as you can (stretching the hamstring). Then move the same leg backward as far as possible (stretching the iliopsoas). Move only from the hip joint, not the waist. Repeat this a few times. Roll over and do the movement on the other side.

11. Let the hip fall forward. Return to the middle and let it fall backward. Repeat a few times, alternating sides.

12. Lift your head up and let it fall behind the arm. Lift head up from your extended arm and let it fall in front of the arm. Repeat a few times alternating sides. This is a good stretch for the neck muscles.

13. Roll over onto your stomach. Place your hands on the floor in front of your face, palms down and elbows bent. Rest your head on your hands.

14. Bend your knees and flop your lower legs from side to side. Play and enjoy this movement.

15. On your stomach, bend the knees and let your legs fall apart and together.

16. On your stomach bend your knees and lift one knee, then the other, towards the ceiling. Move only from the hip joint, not from the waist, to not strain the back.

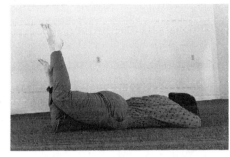

16.

17. On your stomach straighten both legs and raise one at a time towards the ceiling. Alternate. Be careful to again move only from the hip.

18. On your stomach lift and lower one elbow at a time. Move the elbow freely in a dance. This movement loosens up the shoulder blade connections to the neck and trunk.

19. On your stomach roll your head side to side, forehead on hands, without effort. This loosens the muscles that connect the head and neck.

20. Leave your head on the floor and move your arms straight out to the side, palms down. Lift up one shoulder at a time. Alternate a few times. This moves the whole shoulder girdle.

21. Again, with your forehead on the floor, bend your elbows at right angles. From the elbow, lift the hand and forearm only toward the ceiling and alternate, in the Cleopatra position. Feel the back of your neck while you move, specifically for the dowager hump.

22. Come up on your knees with your head down, arms stretched out forward in front of you, hands on the floor. Stretch, sitting back on your heels.

23. Bend your elbows. Place your weight on your forearms and lower leg. Rock forward and backward, loosening up the lower back and hip joint.

24. On hands and knees, sway your seat from side to side.

25. On hands and knees, move your seat to the right side and sit down. Lift up, move to the middle, move your seat to the left side, and sit down. Alternate.

26. Prepare to stand. Place the balls and toes of your feet on the floor and push off, raising your seat up in the air until your legs are straight. Walk towards your hands with your head down. Slowly come up, all the way to standing. Your head should be the last to come up.

27. Lift your arms up to the sides for a deep breath!

Any movements on the floor involving the legs influence the lower back. Freeing the leg in the hip joint allows movement into the back. Doing these exercises with ease can correct improperly carried weight over the pelvis (either too far forward or too far backward).

Hip Joint and Lower Back: the Cable Car Driver

The lying-down partner is passive in all the movements, allowing his limbs to be moved, exerting no effort. The standing partner is active.

1. The partners face each other. One lies down, and the other is stationed first at her partner's feet, then at his head.

2. Standing partner: lift up both his legs by the ankles and rest them on your waist, swaying side to side.

3. Step back, holding your partner's legs in your hands, and swing his legs side to side.

4. Returning to the center, lower one leg down to your side, bending slightly at the waist. Alternate four times.

5. Push both legs straight up towards his head as far as possible without hurting your partner, keeping his legs straight at the knee to stretch his lower back. Repeat three times.

6. Hold both legs up with one hand and walk around your partner until you are standing behind his head. His legs now straddle his head.

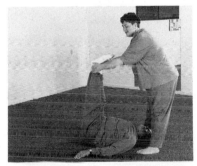

7.

7. Grasp his ankles and pull both legs towards you by leaning backwards. Repeat three or four times.

8. With his legs still over his head, alternately pull each leg toward you like a cable car driver. The standing person is the driver who works her arms and hips backward and forward to move

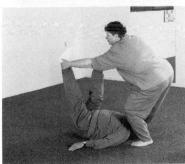

8.

the lever of the cable car. The legs are like the lever of the cable car. The partner on the floor receives the movements as the lever moves forward and backward.

9. Then pull both legs towards you to lift his seat. Continue this movement and swing his lifted seat side to side. Do not go any further than is enjoyable for your partner on the floor.

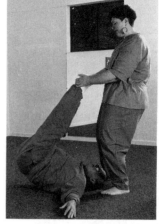

9.

11. Walk around to the original position facing away from your partner. The floor partner now bends his knees with his feet toward the ceiling. The standing partner can sit on his feet, to be bounced gently up and down. The floor partner then pushes the sitting partner off his feet to standing and lowers his feet to the floor.

This sequence stretches the hamstrings, lower back and *gluteus* muscles, and it mobilizes the sacroiliac. If these movements are done gently they are very pleasurable and will not hurt the neck, shoulders or back.

The Hip Joint and Lower Back: the Bicycle

Please follow the directions carefully in order to get the maximum benefit from these seemingly easy movements. They are intended to loosen the hip joints, lower back and hamstrings. These easy movements prepare you for a fairly vigorous stretch at the end.

1. Partners lie on their backs, both feet touching and legs together.

2. Roll your feet and legs side to side to the beat of the music. Feel the rotation in the hip joint.

3. Come up on your elbows while still moving.

4. Straighten your arms while still moving.

5. Stretch forward and hold your partner's right hand. Keep turning your feet with knees straight.

6. Stretch forward and hold your partner's left hand. Keep turning your feet with knees straight.

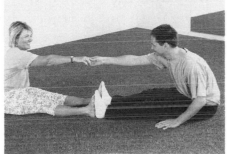

5.

7. Stretch forward and hold both hands. Keep turning your feet with knees straight.

8. Let go and lie down on your back.

9. Feet touching and legs apart, turn your feet toward and away from each other.

10. Come up on your elbows, still moving feet.

11. Straighten your arms, still moving feet.

12. Reach forward and hold right hands, still moving feet.

13. Reach forward and hold left hands, still moving feet.

14. Reach forward and hold both hands, still moving feet.

15. Let go and rest.

16. Lie on your back; bend knees with soles of feet touching each other.

17. Bicycle motion forward and backward to the beat of the music.

18. Continue bicycling; come up on elbows.

19. Continue bicycling; straighten arms.

20. Sit up completely. Bend knees out, feet on the floor with toes touching. Hold your partner's hands and lean forward and backward, slowly at first.

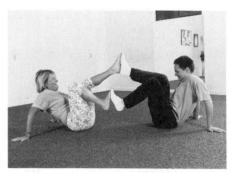

19.

21. Increase the momentum, rocking until one partner is lying down on the floor and the other rocks forward and lifts her seat slightly off the floor. Repeat three times, exchanging positions (Rocking Horse).

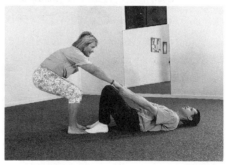

21.

22. Continue the momentum until one partner is standing while the other is lying down. Alternate six times.

23. Finally, one partner remains standing and pulls the other person up too.

Lots of fun to do at the end of class. High energy, works the whole spine.

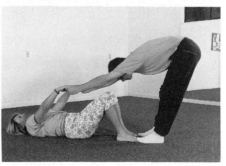

22.

Climbing the Wall Upside-Down

1. Find a spot by the wall where you can lie with your seat against the wall and your legs straight up in the air and against the wall.

2. Lift your seat up, starting with your legs low, and walk up the wall a bit. Slowly let your seat sink, vertebra by vertebra, feeling a stretch in your neck.

3. Walk your legs up the wall, again lifting your seat. Both legs should remain straight. Lower the right leg over your head towards your nose. Alternate legs and then walk down gradually, vertebra by vertebra.

4. Rest.

5. Bend your knees with your feet flat against the wall. Walk a few steps up the wall. Lift up your seat as far as you can and then lower it. Repeat two times. Lift up again, this time lifting each hip alternately, one side at a time. Repeat and lower.

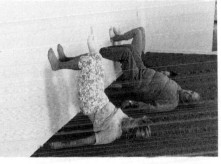
5.

6. Stretch your arms out to the side. With your legs straight up against the wall, roll your head slowly from side to side.

7. Stretch your arms out to the side. Now move your right hand across your chest, reaching as far as possible towards the left. Return your right arm to your right side by sliding the hand along the arm and across the chest. Repeat, alternating sides a few times.

8. Rest. Lower your knees to your chest.

9. Walk your legs up the wall. Raise your head off the floor. Reach towards your left toes with your right arm. Alternate. Lower your head to the floor each time you change sides.

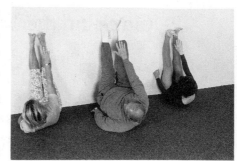

9.

10. Lift your seat way up, until your weight is on your shoulders. Place your hands under your hips for support. Extend one leg straight backwards behind you, then the other. Slowly alternate your legs, back and forth like a scissors.

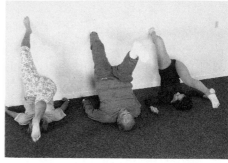

10.

11. Bring both legs together, and lower them over your head into the plow.

12. Slowly lower them back down again and rest. Bend your knees and lower your hips to the floor.

13. Roll over to one side.

14. Continue over onto your hands and knees. Very s-l-o-w-l-y come up to a standing position and reach up, hands and arms extending high into the air, into a big stretch.

This is a useful way to work your back and to mobilize the legs, hips, and trunk. It moves the whole spine and encourages free head movement from side to side. The weight of the upper torso is supported, allowing the hips to move further.

Pelvic-Leg Connection: the Grapevine

The following steps are a Greek circle dance called the grapevine.

1. Hold hands in a circle.

2. Step forward and backward with the right leg. Start slowly, half time to the music, and then move twice as fast. Repeat with the left leg.

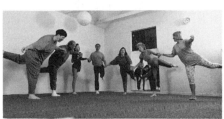

4.

3. Lift the right leg up and step forward, bend the knee as you put your foot down, lift the right leg up, and return to the middle. Repeat with the left leg.

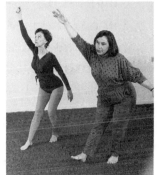

5.

4. Lift the right leg backward and step backward. Lift the right leg up and return to the middle. Repeat with the left leg.

5. Put the right leg forward and left leg back. Rock the hip forward and back several times with your feet on the ground. Movement is in the hip joint. Repeat with the legs reversed.

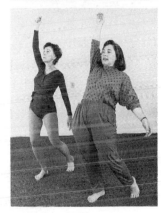

5.

6. Lift the right leg straight forward and return to the center. Lift the left leg straight back and return to the center. Repeat a few times and reverse legs. Now increase the momentum, letting the upper body lean forward and backward, rocking like a seesaw over

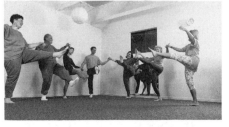

6.

the hip joint several times.

7. Turn one foot out to the side, return to the center, then turn out the other foot. Repeat several times alternating feet, then moving twice as fast.

8. Place one foot out to the side and turn the whole leg inwards on the ball of the foot. Repeat several times alternating legs, then speed up the tempo to twice as fast.

9. Lift one knee and lower it. Lift the other knee and lower it several times. Alternate, and then move twice as fast.

9.

10. Lift one leg straight up and forward into the center of the circle. Alternate legs a few times.

11. Lift one leg straight backward and up. Alternate legs a few times. RAISE THE LEG IN BACK ONLY FROM THE HIP JOINT. DO NOT FORCE YOUR LOWER BACK!

12. Without holding hands, bend forward at hip joint, knees bent and rest hands on your mid thighs. Wiggle your seat from side to side.

13. In the same position, alternately bend and straighten the knee.

14. In the same position, move both knees side to side, rolling over the feet. The movement is in the ankle.

15. Return to standing.

16. Step to the side and return to the center. Alternate.

17. Step forward across the body, step to the side, step backward across the body, step to the side.

18. Hold hands in a circle for balance. Lift the right leg to the side and raise it in a half circle across the front of the body to the other side and then bring it back to the side. Repeat with the other leg.

19. Hold hands and move the leg to the side. Lift the leg up and move it in a half circle in back of the body to the other side, and then circle it back. Repeat with the other leg.

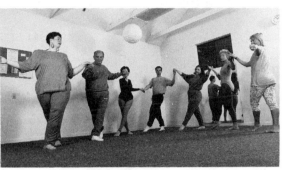

18.

20. Still standing in a circle, continue to hold hands. Combine the last two movements by swinging the right leg forward, across the body. Touch the toes to the floor and return the leg across the front of the body. Continue around behind you, completing almost a full circle. The foot touches the ground then returns to the side. Repeat with the left leg.

21. Raise the right leg forward and across the body and then lower it to the floor. The left leg steps to the same side. Move the right leg sideways and then backwards and across. The left leg steps to the same side. Move the right leg forward and across. Keep going around the circle. Switch direction. Now the left leg steps forward and across; the right leg steps to the same side. Bring the left leg backward and across; the right leg steps to the same side. Go once around the circle in each direction. Do this in varied tempos from slow to fast.

This sequence uses all the possible movements of the hip joint. The circular movements of the legs work all the muscle connections between the legs, the floor of the pelvis and the hip joints, easily loosening them up. This helps loosen the lower back and sacroiliac joint.

Waltz Tempo Sequence across the Floor

1. Partners walk across the floor side by side, letting their arms swing freely.

2. Add a waltz step (1, 2, 3 – 1, 2, 3) and swing both arms out to the same side. Don't hold hands.

3. Continuing the waltz step and arm swing, lift the leg out to the opposite side of the arm swing.

4. Holding hands for balance, swing the leg out to the side and across in front of the body in a circular motion. Alternate.

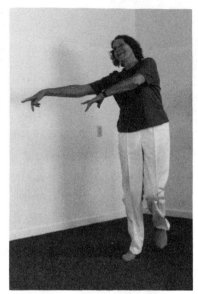

2.

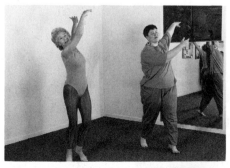

2.

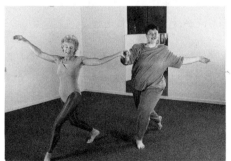

4.

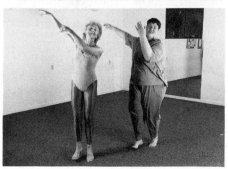

2.

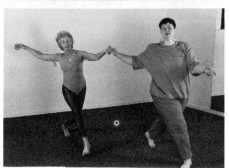

4.

90

5. Let go of hands. Swing the arms to one side and legs to the opposite side, beginning a figure-eight motion with the arms.

6. Move the arms in a figure eight while lifting the leg backwards as we continue to move forward.

7. Turn around. Hold your partner's hand. Lift your leg backward and take a waltz step backwards (lift – step, lift – step).

8. Stand side by side. Hold your partner's inside hand. Swing the arm you are holding forward and backward, while waltzing across the floor.

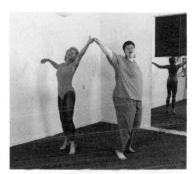

9.

9. Continuing to waltz, turn away from your partner while holding one hand.

10. Continuing to waltz, turn toward your partner while holding one hand.

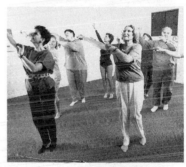

11.

11. Do it again with abandonment! Let yourself dance.

These basic movements are played with and varied, with different tempos and different routines. They are designed to loosen up the body and bring forth the joy of movement. The point of the waltz is to feel the joy of moving while loosening the shoulder girdle, chest and hip joint.

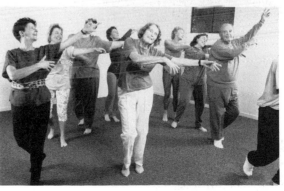

11.

91

Suggested Music

"Stardust," Willie Nelson, CBS Records.
    Side 1: "Stardust," "Georgia on my Mind"
    Side 2: "On the Sunny Side of the Street," "Don't Get Around Much Anymore"

"Elite Hotel," Emmy Lou Harris, Reprise Records
    Side 1: "Together Again," "Feeling Single Seein' Double," "One of These Days"

"The Manhattan Transfer," Atlantic Records
    Side 2: "Java Jive," "Occapella"

"The Sting," Sound Track, MCA Records
    Side 1: "Solace," "The Entertainer"

"The Mills Brothers Great Hits," Dot Records
    Side 2: "Lazy River," "Be My Life's Companion"

"Nat King Cole," EMI Records
    Side 1: "Don't Blame Me," "Sometimes I'm Happy"
    Side 2: "When I Grow Too Old to Dream," "Exactly Like You"

"Silver Wings," Mike Rowland, Music Design, Inc.
    Side 1: "L'apocalypse des Animaux"

Vangelis Papathamssiou, Polydor Records
    Side 1: "La Petite Fille de la Mer"

"Song of the Seashore," James Galway, RCA Records
    Side A: "Song of the Seashore"
    Side B: "Song of the Seashell," "My Homeland"

"Path of Joy," Daniel Kobialka, Li-sem Enterprises
    Side 1: "Jesu, Joy of Man's Desiring"

"Zamfir," Mercury Pan Flute: Gheorghe Zamfir
    Side B: "The Lonely Shepherd," "Black Rose," "Theme from Sum-

mer of '42," "Bilitis"

"White Winds," Andreas Vollenweider, CBS Records
    Side 1: "Hall of the Stairs"
    Side 2: "Phases of the Three Moons," "Flight Feet," "Trilogy"

"Recycling the Blues," Taj Mahal, Columbia Records
    Side 2: "Cakewalk into Town"

"Moonstruck," Sound track, Capitol Records
    Side 2: "Musetta's Waltz," "Canzone per Loretta," "Moonglow"

"Legend," Bob Marley, Island Records
    Side 1: "Could You Be Loved," "Three Little Birds"
    Side 2: "Jamming"

"The Harder They Come," Jimmy Cliff, Sound Track, Island Records
    Side 1: "Draw Your Brakes," "Rivers of Babylon," "The Harder
    They Come"

"Steppin," The Pointer Sisters, ABC Records
    Side 1: "How Long"
    Side 2: "Save the Bones for Henry Jones"

"Thriller," Michael Jackson, Epic Records (CBS)
    Side 1: "Wanna Be Startin' Something'"
    Side 2: "Billie Jean"

"Chronicle," The Staple Singers, Stax Records
    Side 1: "Respect Yourself," "I'll Take You There"

"The Changer and the Changed," Olivia Records
    Side 1: "Song of the Soul"

"Prisoner in Disguise," Linda Ronstadt, Electra Records
    Side 1: "Love Is A Rose," "Roll Um Easy"

"Night Songs," Earl Klugh, Capitol Records
    Side 1: "Look of Love," "Nature Boy"
    Side 2: "Night Song," "C.C. Rider," "Shadow of Your Smile"

"Deep Breakfast," Ray Lynch, Music West Records
    Side 1: "Celestial Soda Pop," "Falling in the Garden"
    Side 2: "Rhythm in the Pews"

SUGGESTED MUSIC

"The Pachelbel Canon," Maurice André, R.C.A. Records
  Side A: "Canon in D"
"I Heard It Through The Grapevine," Marvin Gaye, Motown Records
"From Branch to Branch," Leon Redbone, Emerald City Records
  Side 1: "Mamas Got a Baby Named TeNaNa," "Seduced"
  Side 2: "Why," "My Blue Heaven," "Prairie Lullaby"
"Banish Misfortune," Malcolm Dalglish, June Appal Records
  Side 1: "Sir John Fenwick"
"Old Time Music With Fiddle and Guitar," Clark Kessinger, Rounder
  Records
  Side 1: "When I Grow To Old To Dream," "Tennessee Waltz"
  Side 2: "The Waltz You Saved For Me," "Good Night Waltz"
"Bordertown," Bennie Wallace, Blue Note Records
  Side 1: "Stormy Weather"
  Side 2: "Bordertown," "Dance With A Dolly"

Rosen Method Training

Rosen Method workshops and certification training programs are offered in the United States, Canada, Europe and the USSR. They are co-ordinated by the following centers. For information contact:

Northeast and Canada: Sue Brenner (510) 653-9113

Rocky Mountain area and Southwest: Sandra Wooten (510) 845-9613

West Coast: Nancy Powell (510) 845-6606

Scandinavia: Axelson's Gymnastika Institute
Gastrikegatan 10-12
11334 Stockholm, Sweden

USSR: Salus International Health Institute
Attention: Mary Kay Wright Malear
16 Bolotnikorskaya
Moscow, 113149 USSR
Phone: 110-33-76
USA phone: (510) 254-9377